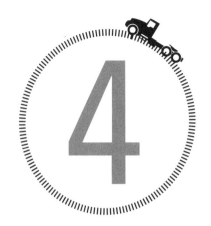

Minute Fit

The Metabolism Accelerator for the
Time Crunched, Deskbound,
and **Stressed-Out**

Siphiwe Baleka
"America's Fittest Trucker"
with L. Jon Wertheim

TOUCHSTONE | New York London Toronto Sydney New Delhi

Contents

Introduction

What you're about to read is a take on weight loss unlike any other
ever created, one built on real-world experience and proven effective
on the most weight-challenged population in the world. Because I'm
not a nutritionist or a weight-loss guru or a TV host peddling a new
diet trend or a crazy new exercise fad.

I'm a truck driver.

You might say that I'm at ground zero for the obesity war. For the
last decade, I've worked in the long-haul trucking industry, statistically
the least healthy occupation in America and the line of work with the
highest incidence of obesity. I've seen firsthand how obesity ravages a
body, diminishes a life, erodes self-confidence, and ultimately kills. I've
worked alongside people who believe they have no control over their
lives, who long ago resigned themselves to irreversible weight gain and
early death.

You see, truck drivers might be a unique breed, but the challenges
they face are the same that most of us face: too much driving, too
much sitting, and too many bad food choices. And you don't have to
be locked into a cross-country haul to experience the damaging ef-

fects of the driver's seat. In fact, a 2016 study in *The Lancet Diabetes & Endocrinology*, a British medical journal, found that those of us who drive to work weigh more and have a higher percentage of body fat than those who get back and forth by other methods—including even public transportation.

In fact, those of us who drive more than thirty minutes each way to work can pack on an extra 15 pounds every two years, say researchers. Sitting is bad for us for a number of reasons, but one of them is because it decreases our levels of LPL (lipoprotein lipase), a fat-burning enzyme secreted by the large muscles in our legs. It also damages our bone density while raising overall blood pressure, putting our muscles, our hearts, and even our brains at risk.

The stereotype is that people who spend all that time on their butts do it because they're not motivated. But that's simply not true; the reality is that most of us work really hard, and nowadays working hard means being locked into a seated position.

And all that hard work is doing us damage. Consider this: A Cleveland Clinic study found that since 1995, the average age of people suffering potentially deadly heart attacks has dropped from age sixty-four down to age sixty, and 40 percent of those heart attacks can be linked to obesity. High blood pressure, diabetes, and chronic obstructive pulmonary disease are the primary contributors, the researchers said. Another study found that people who sit for six hours a day or more are 40 percent more likely to die over the next fifteen years than those who sit for less than three hours a day. And a 2016 study in the *American Journal of Preventive Medicine* found that about 4 percent of all deaths can be attributed directly to spending too much time on our butts.

It's ironic: We live at a time when it's never been easier to live healthy. Restaurants give us calorie counts for the food we're about to order. We wear watches on our wrists that track how many steps we walk during a day and the quality of our sleep. Everywhere you look, there's a new gym, fitness center, or a yoga studio. Yet, overall, obesity rates have never been higher.

Maybe, up until now, you've been one of those people fighting—and losing—the battle against fat. Chances are, you're unhappy with how you look. Disappointed in your energy levels. Worried about the creeping health threats presented by your expanding weight, from back pain to diabetes to heart disease. Frustrated by the impact it's had on your quality of life, from limited flexibility to a lackluster sex drive.

And maybe, like many of us, you've tried different methods to try to get back some control—fad diet plans, exercise routines, and specialty health foods that do little more than make your life miserable, whittling away your time, money, and energy while having only the slightest impact on your weight.

I've proven that fact time and time again with the 4-Minute Fit, a program I developed that has worked for thousands of truckers—stripping away 20, 40, even 60 pounds or more in a matter of just months, without specialty foods, without hunger or deprivation, without long hours in the gym.

Because here's the reality: our war against obesity is winnable. The conflict is preventable. The problem is solvable. The damage is reversible. The epidemic can be thwarted. And, unlike most wars, we have all the power. If we're determined to put up a fight and sustain our attack, the opponent is helpless. If we use the resources and technology at our disposal, we will prevail.

The 4-Minute Fit is a remarkably easy and effective plan, one that requires you to exercise at high intensity for just four minutes a day—and up to a maximum of no more than fifteen minutes a day—and to eat a protein meal or snack every three hours. That's it. The 4-Minute

Fit works by targeting your hormonal system, boosting your metabolism, and forcing your body to burn fat for energy.

And this plan works for people whose weight-loss challenges are just like yours, except worse. We're talking about a subset of Americans who spend their day sitting—sometimes for eight, ten, twelve hours at a stretch—and then sitting again the next day and the day after that. Who can't get to a gym because they're always on the road. Who don't often have access to a kitchen or traditional "health food" because their meals are often limited to truck stops and fast-food joints. Who don't always get consistent sleep because they're slaves to their trucking schedules.

Bottom line: if this plan works for the people with the most severe weight-loss challenges, it can, and will, work for you.

The 4-Minute Fit is the fast, simple, effective method that works for anybody. There are no complicated formulas. No expensive equipment is required. Your level of education doesn't matter. If you're comfortable with basic digital technology, there are smartphone apps that can help you make the plan even more automatic. But if not, no worries: the old school will work just fine. And it *will* work for you: Whether you're an aspiring twentysomething or well settled into middle age. Whether you have a sedentary job or an active job. Whether you're a millionaire or you're broke. Whether you're time crunched or have all day to fill. You can do this!

The 4-Minute Fit is a carb-control eating plan that gives you the power to cut down, slowly, on the foods that contribute most to our weight gain, while increasing your intake of delicious foods (even stuff like burgers, ribs, and hot wings). All the while, you'll be flattening your belly, shedding those extra rolls, and enjoying a calmer, saner, simpler life. This incredibly easy-to-follow plan, combined with a metabolism-boosting workout that takes just minutes a day, will make such a shocking, rapid, and dramatic difference in your body, you'll be stunned by the results. It all boils down to seven simple strategies:

The Seven Strategies

1. No matter what, get fifteen minutes of exercise a day, every day.

2. Each workout must include at least four minutes of vigorous activity.

3. Work multiple muscle groups at the same time.

4. Always eat after a workout.

5. Eat breakfast. Then eat something every three hours.

6. Keep healthy snacks within reach.

7. Log your nutrition and fitness.

That's it. With this plan you will spike your metabolism and force your body to burn fat.

1   My Personal Weight-Loss Journey

No life-improvement plan is going to be effective for you unless you believe in it, and one of the keys to believing in a system is holding trust in the leader. A sports team that doesn't have faith in the coach is in trouble. Same for the company whose employees are skeptical of the CEO. So before we get started, let me tell you a little about me and the strange path that led me from Yale University to the life of a truck driver.

Just about every trucker has a rich backstory. You see, truckers come in all shapes and sizes, all shades and age groups. We come from all over America and beyond, from small towns for sure, but also from cities. We're men and we're also women. We're married and divorced, straight and gay, grandmothers in their sixties and bachelors in their twenties. We come from all different kinds of education levels, hold a wide array of political and religious values, and enjoy a diverse pool of interests outside of work.

For a guy like me who's hopelessly, incurably outgoing, this diversity is one of the great pluses of the job. I love this aspect. One day you're talking to a Native American from New Mexico who's telling you about his tribal rituals; the next day you're talking with a former hippie from Maine who writes poetry whenever her motor is turned off.

My story? I've had a lot of adventures. I've been to dozens of foreign countries under all sorts of different circumstances. I went to college at Yale but have worked with street gangs in Chicago and been part of the squatters' movement in Europe.

There's been love and loss and lots of passion. There's been uncertainty—times when I haven't been sure where I was going to sleep or how I was going to eat. There have been triumphs—from becoming the first African American to be named an All-Ivy League swimmer, to being named America's Fittest Trucker. And like you, I've had my share of disappointments as well.

My birth name was Anthony Blake. I grew up in the far west suburbs of Chicago, a patch of heartland suburbia built on the fields of a long-fallow farm. My parents split up when I was a young boy, and I was the rare African American kid who was brought up by a single father.

Like an omnivore that eats everything, as a kid, I played all sports. There was always a ball or mitt or tennis racket attached to my arm. But I took a particular interest in swimming. I wasn't big or even graceful, but I loved technique, finding little ways to improve, always tinkering to uncover tricks that could make me faster and more efficient. I loved to compete and test myself against others who were also trying their hardest. By age ten, I was an Illinois state champion in swimming. As a teenager I had a national ranking.

An uncle of mine by marriage, Hayes Jones, had won a gold medal in hurdling in the 1964 Olympic Games in Tokyo. I talked to him once about all that he had achieved in sports and what he had to do to get there. I remember that I didn't come away awed or feeling like I had been talking to a superhero. I came away thinking, Well, hey, he did it. Why not me, too?

I had always done well in school academically, and so I was fortunate that when it was time to pick a college I had plenty of choices. I settled on Yale, largely for the swimming program. Yale had once been an absolute swimming powerhouse, winning four NCAA titles over eleven years.

Unfortunately, that span was from 1942 to 1953. (In fact, under Coach Robert J. H. Kiphuth, Yale had 528 wins and just 12 losses during those eleven years, for the greatest collegiate winning percentage of any sports team in history.) But I arrived on campus full of optimism, convinced that I could help the program get back to greatness and excited about working under Yale's terrific longtime coach, Frank Keefe.

Since my early childhood, I've always liked going against convention. I didn't rebel for the sake of rebelling, but I never minded being different. And my time at Yale just highlighted that fact. I didn't mind that most of the best swimmers were from California and Florida, and here I was, from the guts of Illinois. Or that most other swimmers, including my teammates, were tall and lanky and classically built, while I was just 5 foot 8 and maybe 140 pounds, soaking wet. While swimmers were supposed to specialize in a single event, I was a generalist, who swam sprints but also swam long distances. I wasn't going to worry about whether I fit in; I was going to trust my work ethic and my techniques and my desire and drive to succeed.

At the time, there had yet to be an African American swimmer in the Olympics, and there was still a great deal of mindless prejudice against African Americans in the sport. One of the most memorable moments of my teenage years came when a baseball executive named Al Campanis went on national television and, without a trace of embarrassment or self-consciousness, said, "Why are black men, or black people, not good swimmers? Because they don't have the buoyancy."

If that's the way most of America thought of black people, well, I was going to change all that.

Early in my freshman year at Yale, I was placed in a pool lane with a senior, Andrew Geller, who was the best swimmer on the team. Frustrated that he wasn't swimming fast enough for my liking, I passed him, which was considered poor pool etiquette, especially for an incoming freshman. He was furious and let me know it. I shot back, "I don't care who you are, if you aren't going fast enough, I'm going in front of you." That pretty much summed up who I was at the time.

By my sophomore year, I had placed fifth in the Eastern Seaboard Swim Championships and made the all-conference team, becoming the first African American swimmer ever to be named to the All-Ivy League team. That year Yale finished 10–3. My junior season, the team was 9–1.

And then my life took a sharp turn. I went to the US Open meet, my opportunity to qualify for the US Olympic Trials in the 100-meter freestyle event. Looking back, I might have been a long shot. But failure hadn't really crossed my mind. It rarely did back then. This was just something I needed to do before I could make the US Olympic team.

Except that my expectations outstripped my abilities. Well, you can guess what happened: I missed qualifying for the Olympic Trials by less than a second. Eight-tenths of a second, to be exact, or about as much time as it takes to read the words *eight tenths*.

I knew that this had been my one chance for the Olympics, and it wasn't going to happen. There was no arguing, no do-overs, no one I could appeal to. The data—in this case, the electronic timer—had said that I had failed. I remember standing in the cool-down pool in Minneapolis and crying, my tears mixing with the chlorinated pool water. I was crying over a dream that had died. But I was also crying for something bigger: my attitude, competitive streak, and technique simply hadn't been enough to get me through.

I returned to Yale for my senior year, but I didn't want to swim anymore. The quest was over, and I was heartbroken. So much so that one evening, a few of my roommates found me passed out near a bottle of pills, and I spent a few days in the psych ward of Yale–New Haven

Hospital. It was the first time I had really wanted something and didn't accomplish it. And that was a shock to the system. I wasn't released until I could convince the doctors I wasn't a danger to myself.

As part of my recovery program, I got back in the pool and started swimming again. Late in my senior year, I helped Yale win a share of the Ivy League title for the first time in years. That was on a Saturday night. On Monday morning, I was gone.

Graduation was only a few weeks away, and I was in good academic standing. But I felt like I had gotten all I could out of school. I was tired of reading about Jesus and Buddha and all these other spiritual luminaries who had followed their destinies. I wanted to do it, experience the world for myself. So I hitchhiked home, dropped off some bags, and told my dad what I had done. He was less than pleased, as you might guess, and tried to talk me out of it. But it was too late. I told him, "I'm going to travel the world. I don't know when I'll be back, if ever." And then I headed off.

I spent the next fifteen years traveling, following my heart. I surfed in California and hitchhiked in Europe. I threaded my way from Amsterdam to Prague to Trinidad to Honduras to Togo to Ethiopia. There wasn't much in the way of a long-term plan or organizing principle, just a deep sense that life needed to be experienced and an unshakable belief that it would all work out.

People often ask me if I ever finished college and got my Yale degree. The answer, I'm happy to say, is yes. It was a goal that I set and—after working harder than I thought—I was able to accomplish. When I was in my mid-twenties, after a few years of wandering, I decided to re-enroll. I was so close to graduating that I had to finish, and Yale—which wants as many of its students as possible to finish with a degree—let me back in. One problem: I felt like I couldn't bother my father with tuition; I had put him through enough. But after paying for classes, I had nothing left to pay for room and board. But I was determined, so I did what I had to do.

I had recently been in Europe and had joined the squatters' movement there. I thought, Why don't I try that here? I spent that final semester of college living rent-free in abandoned buildings and in the swim team locker room, eating most of my meals at the local soup kitchens. It was hardly the fun and easy college life that other kids were living. It was the opposite, in fact. But I finally got that degree.

As my thirtieth birthday approached, I decided to go back to Africa. Like a lot of African Americans, I felt as though I didn't really know my personal history. Connecting with my ancestral heritage became very important to me. I traveled all over the continent, mostly using money I had saved or earning it along the way by making wood furniture. In South Africa, I met with tribal elders. They said that when a son of the soil returns home, he should get a new name. They gave me the name Siphiwe (pronounced seh-PEA-way), a name common among the Xhosa and Zulu tribes. They said it means "Gift of the Creator." For a last name, they chose Baleka, an anagram of A. Blake. It means "Fast" and "He Who Had Escaped."

By my mid-thirties, though, I was tired of having no real plan and no real income. I knew I wasn't cut out for a corporate job. (Besides, I may have had a Yale degree, but to say that my résumé was "nontraditional" was an understatement.) There was essentially a fifteen-year gap in my work history, one that wasn't going to be easy to explain to a corporate recruiter.

A truck driver friend named Jaberi made a suggestion to me: Drive a truck. It suits your nomadic lifestyle. You got plenty of time to think, and you can save a lot of money. I did what I usually do and said, "Why not? I'll try it." I traveled to southern Missouri and enrolled in Prime's uniquely successful Student Driver Program. I got my commercial driver's license, spent another four or five months on the road with an instructor-driver, and eventually became a lease operator.

The job fed something in me and suited my personality. The roads are a wilderness, each trip a unique adventure. But, unlike my previous adventures, this one brought steady employment and a plan. I didn't mind the solitude. And driving triggered this feeling of familiarity. I hadn't really been in a pool since I'd left Yale, but here I was maneuvering in a lane, reaching a destination, and then returning to where I started in the opposite lane; getting lost inside my head; feeling a sense of independence as I paced myself. The parallels between driving and swimming were hard to miss.

And I liked the unpredictability, too. One week, I'd be hauling flank steak to the West Coast. The next week, I'd be transporting diapers to Miami. You just never knew where you were headed, what part of the country you'd see next, what kind of weather and air you'd be experiencing. But to me, that was all part of the fun. So, too, was gaining an understanding of how important my new job really was. So many of our daily necessities—clothes, food, furniture, medicine—come, literally, off the back of a truck. Drive a truck for a little while, and you soon realize you're a vital part of the economy. Without truck drivers crisscrossing highways and delivering goods we use every day, this country doesn't run. It's that simple.

But here's what I didn't like: the changes to my body. For all the adventures I'd had over the years, one of my most vivid moments—a real plot point in my life—came when I realized that I didn't like how I looked.

In less than two months on the job, I had somehow managed to gain more than 10 percent of my body weight. At that rate, I could come close to doubling my body weight within a year. My energy level was low. It almost felt like I was wearing a costume—one that I couldn't take off at the end of the day. It wasn't just that I didn't like what I saw when I looked in the mirror; it's that I didn't even recognize the figure in front of me. *Hey, wait a second: This isn't what I look like. Is it? Really?*

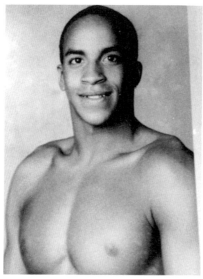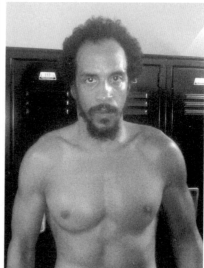

Yale swim team photo — Starting to let myself go

This was all a new sensation for me, almost like visiting a foreign country. See, for my entire life, I had put a premium on health and fitness and, yeah, I'll admit it, on my looks. I had always been an athlete. Over the years, I had struggled with plenty of concerns and challenges. But fitting into my clothes had never been one of them.

Now? All that muscle, originally built up from so many sessions in the weight room and countless nautical miles in the pool, was atrophying. My abs were turning into flab. I lost my beloved six-pack and picked up love handles instead. I even felt my face stretching out and feeling heavier on my neck.

And maybe worse still, there was a real price that came with all this, physically and psychologically. I felt sluggish. My energy was low. I was moody. This unwanted weight gain was affecting everything from my sleep to my sex life.

I looked around and saw my new coworkers. Don't get me wrong. They were—and are—absolutely fantastic people. But they were also, for the most part, overweight and not on a path to live a long life.

There are 3.5 million truckers in the United States. A full 86 percent of them are overweight, and nearly 70 percent are obese, the highest proportion of any profession in America. A recent Gallup Healthways analysis revealed that transportation workers, including truck drivers, have the highest risk for chronic health problems of any occupation in America. The Centers for Disease Control and Prevention (CDC) put long-haul trucking at the top of the list for jobs with the highest rates of obesity. If you wanted to find one profession that embodied the country's obesity epidemic, this one, sadly, would be it. Trucking is at the heart of this national crisis.

How bad is it? As I write this, the overall life expectancy for the US population is 78.7 years. For truckers who own their own vehicles, it's 55.7 years; for union drivers, it's 63 years. Some of this is directly because of the obesity and bad health that runs rampant in the industry. It's also because of indirect effects. Bad habits, erratic hours, and sleep deprivation lead to the factors that cause fatal traffic accidents on the roads.

Bottom line: I love driving, but not at the expense of my health. And certainly not at the expense of my life.

This low moment was followed by what you might call an aha moment. I was at home watching TV one night, wallowing in my new weight gain, when an infomercial came on. It was for something called the ROM Machine. ROM stands for "range of motion," and it was a giant contraption that promised the users the benefits of sixty minutes of cardio, thirty minutes of strength training, and twenty minutes of stretching in—get this—a four-minute workout. I was like, *Come on, really? Four minutes? This is a joke, right?* I'm watching athlete after athlete on the screen—this parade of smiling, buff-looking, muscle-bound guys—get on this machine and say that after four minutes, they're exhausted. Just dog-tired. It's the hardest workout they've ever done.

As is usually the case with me and infomercials, I'm skeptical. But at the same time, I'm intrigued. A four-minute workout sounds highly questionable, of course. (I mean, that's half the time of eight-minute abs, and people doubted that.) But what I had seen actually made a lot of sense. The machine is like a sit-down bicycle with your legs out in front of you. But there are also handles, and when you pull them, it's as though you're rowing. So it's like you're riding a bike and rowing a boat at the same time. And when you get to the extreme end of the motion, you push back the other way, and the resistance changes. So whether you're pulling or pushing, it's four minutes of maximum resistance, maximum stretch, maximum range of motion. I'm watching this, and the guy in the commercial is explaining the benefits and all the science behind it. He's talking about how, when you use a greater range of muscles over a greater range of motion, you circulate more oxygen, which causes more of the metabolic process to produce energy, which requires fat burning. By the end, I'm thinking that, especially as I'm coming to terms with my new weight gain, this machine would sure help me.

Damn, I want a ROM Machine.

There are two problems.

First, the ROM Machine costs $15,000, which I did not have. In fact, I didn't have much if any money at all at the time. (This is one unfortunate consequence of spending so much of your twenties and early thirties following your bliss.) If it had cost $1.50, I might have needed an installment plan. And second, I am a truck driver, putting thousands of miles on my odometer each week. I can't exactly carry this machine onto my truck.

But I was impressed, and I was inspired. I wasn't going to buy a silly ROM Machine from an infomercial. I started researching the principles behind it. There had to be a way I could start burning fat and shedding all this extra weight without a traditional gym. What I discovered: there *was* a lot of research supporting the idea that a short burst of intense exercise had the same—and sometimes even more—benefits than longer workouts. This came at a time savings, a cost savings, and a reduction in the risk for injury.

Looking back, I see this was the beginning of 4-Minute Fit.

At first there was a lot of trial and even more error. I tried doing exercises that had helped me back when I was swimming competitively—push-ups, sit-ups—but haphazardly, with no plan, no system. I'd pull over at a truck stop or a parking lot, climb out of the cab, get out a piece of cardboard and, right there alongside my truck, get to it. In the beginning, some drivers laughed at me and what I was doing. That was nothing new. Other drivers would say they were looking to lose weight too or that they had once been athletic before their bodies got away from them. But no one asked to join. It was as though they had resigned themselves to being overweight.

Meanwhile, I was determined to lose this weight, but the results weren't coming. At least not fast enough.

Next, I started bringing different types of equipment on the road with me: resistance bands and kettlebells and a weighted vest. Again, it felt good to exercise and sweat a little and get my pulse rate up. But I wasn't seeing the results that I wanted.

Then I tried to get to the next level by experimenting with different exercise programs that were trendy at the time. I did Zumba and P90X and Tae Bo and GSP Rushfit. I would try the DVDs, which wasn't always easy on the road. I'd park the truck on a flat surface and then set up the DVD player so the sun wouldn't create a glare. I would change into workout clothes, connect the DVD to an external speaker so I could hear, and then get in my workout. When I was done, I would have to break everything down, change back into my old clothes, and pack up. My sixty-minute DVD workout was taking more like two hours in total. But I was on a tight schedule—like most of us, including truckers, are—and so I knew that it wasn't going to be sustainable.

I tinkered with my diet, too. I was vegetarian and then pescatarian. I tried Mediterranean and Paleo. I would see results at first, but then inevitably I would slip and the weight would return. Again, when you're pressed for time, you're driving on the interstates, and you're pulling into unfamiliar towns at irregular hours, it's hard to keep to one specific diet.

Adding to this was the difficulty of eating well on the "truckers' grid." See, when you're trucking, assigned to maneuver this steel whale, this fifty-some-foot metal tube weighing as much as 80,000 pounds with cargo, you're mostly staying on interstates. You're not driving to the upmarket parts of town where stores sell grass-fed meat and organic fruits and vegetables. (Honk if you've ever seen a semi parked outside a Whole Foods or Trader Joe's.)

So the challenges I faced were sort of like the challenges we all face, except many times worse. No kitchen, food storage issues . . . If standard diet and fitness plans weren't effective for most of the American population, they certainly weren't going to work for me and my coworkers. I needed something new, a plan that was completely different.

THE START OF A REVOLUTION

Finally, I diagnosed the issue. The problem was one of metabolism. Truck drivers are prime candidates for metabolic syndrome, the medical term for a combination of diabetes, high blood pressure, and obesity that puts you at greater risk of heart disease, stroke, and other conditions affecting blood vessels. If I could figure out a way to boost metabolism while keeping workouts really short (to fit into the hectic schedule) and making eating simple (to compensate for the long hours and shortage of optimal food choices), not only could I change my body, but I could help the men and women who shared the road with me.

A slowing metabolism is the main driver of weight gain for most of us, and among truckers, the problem is even more exaggerated, thanks to our unpredictable schedules. The freight dictates when truckers drive. Sometimes that means driving at night, and sometimes it means driving in the day. It is the rare driver who gets more than six hours of uninterrupted sleep, and it all disrupts circadian rhythms and the natural biological clock. Sleep deprivation accumulates every day, every week, every month, every year that you drive.

And sleep is a major driver of metabolism. The hormones that regulate metabolism—leptin and ghrelin, which control appetite; insulin and adiponectin, which oversee fat storage; human growth factor, which manages muscle; and cortisol and glucagon, which control energy expenditure—are either produced in your sleep or regulated by your sleep patterns. This is a production cycle that is constantly changing and constantly interrupted for truckers. They're not able to produce the hormones properly, so their metabolism doesn't function the way it is supposed to. Again, a huge problem not just for those of us on the road but for anyone who's tied to a desk job and at the mercy of the alarm clock.

But if getting more sleep wasn't an option, what if I tinkered with my metabolism while I was awake? What if I exercised in short bursts? And what if I adjusted my diet—cutting back on carbohydrates and strategically timing protein intake every three hours —an eating strategy that would also help my metabolism to spike?

It was then that I remembered the infomercial, you know, the one for the ROM Machine. They claimed that four minutes a day was all you needed to spike your metabolism and set your body into fat-burning mode. What if I could replicate these same principles when I was on the road? I could do the pulling movement with resistance bands, four minutes, as hard as I can in one direction. And then I could do the pushing by turning it around and doing the movement in the opposite direction. So I would get all the upper-body work that this fancy, expensive ROM Machine would give me, but with the cheap, portable equipment I could afford and fit on my truck. I could take resistance bands on the truck, and I could hook them up

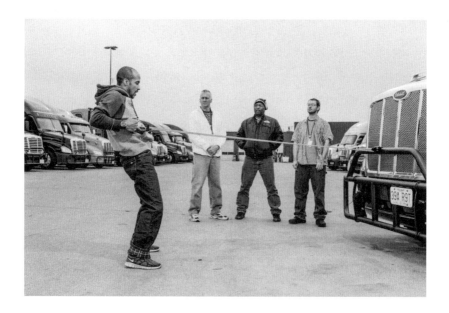

anywhere—to a roadside tree, to the truck, inside the door, or wherever. It was such a complete workout, incorporating just about every group of muscles and working in stretching. And, even better, I could complete the entire routine in just fifteen minutes—the maximum amount of exercise that one should do, for reasons I'll explain in an upcoming chapter.

The results were remarkable. Like a snake molting its skin, I shed the excess weight. I worked myself into the best shape of my adult life and—while still driving full time more than 330 days each year—I returned to competitive swimming. In 2011, I won two events at the US Masters Swimming Spring Nationals and went on to compete in eight sprint and Olympic distance triathlons (winning my age group in two of those races), including the USAT Age Group National Championships. I competed in the 2012 Ironman South Africa, finishing in 214th place out of more than 1,300 athletes. This led one industry magazine to give me the honorary title of the "Fittest Truck Driver in America."

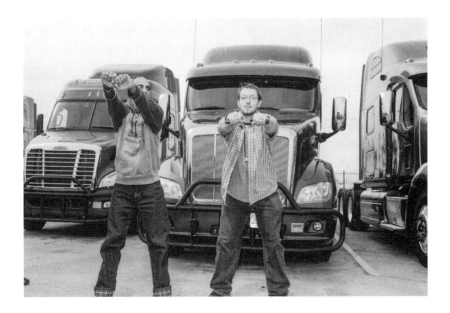

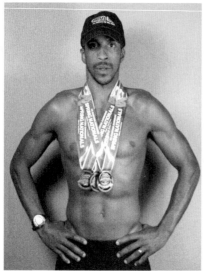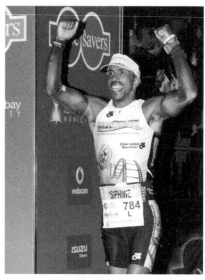

With medals from the 2011 US Masters Swimming Spring Nationals

Crossing the finish line in 214th place at the 2012 Ironman South Africa

I realized something else: the same principles and program that enabled me, in my early forties, to look like the guy above? They could apply to my truck-driving colleagues, too. In fact, the basic principles apply to just about anyone, whether they're obese and looking to cut their BMI in half, or already fit adults who simply wanted to elevate to super-fit.

Now, if I can take a group of sedentary, badly nourished, and exhausted truckers, give them no access to a gym, and *still* strip away enormous amounts of weight while having them exercise just four minutes a day, imagine what I can do for you.

2 How 4 Minutes Can Change Your Life

I've heard a lot of explanations—I don't want to call them excuses—for why people don't exercise or stick to a fitness program. But this is by far the most common: *I don't have time.* People are busy. They have other commitments. Their family is a priority. Or their job or their pets or their DIY projects are a bigger priority. You can imagine the time crunch for truckers, who drive eleven hours during a fourteen-hour period and spend so much of their "free" time working on truck maintenance or filling out all sorts of paperwork. With all these obligations, fitness gets squeezed. *I want to do it, but I just don't have time.* Time is the biggest barrier to exercising consistently.

As a result, the most important component of a successful fitness program is *convenience.* And the easiest way for me to get clients started is to build a program that they can fit into their routine. *You want convenient?* I tell them, All you have to do is move around with maximum intensity for four minutes.

After that the conversation is predictable.

I must have misunderstood you. Four minutes?

Yup, you heard right. Four minutes.

Society has programmed us to think that we need a minimum of thirty to sixty minutes of exercise each day to get any weight-loss results. Most group fitness classes at the gym or health club or YMCA last at least half an hour. Add in the time it takes to get to and from the gym, change clothes, shower, and change clothes again—and you are talking a solid one- to two-hour commitment. Even the home-training programs such as the popular P90X videos average sixty to seventy-five minutes per workout. And that doesn't include setup time and cleanup time.

One consequence of all this: even when we have a block of free time, we assume it's not going to be enough. We have twenty minutes, but in our heads, we have accounted for a thirty-minute workout. So we say, "Nah, I guess it's not happening today. I'll get to it later." But, consciously or subconsciously, we all know that, all too often, later becomes never.

How to Crunch Time

One of the most important determinants affecting exercise adherence is the environmental factor of perceived availability of time. We live in a time-crunched world. Everyone is in a rush. Yet, exercise professionals can assist clients by encouraging the idea that exercise is a priority. Behavioral psychologists have termed the redesigning of beliefs and values "cognitive restructuring." The idea is to replace one line of thinking with another. Instead of "I have too much to do at work today, I'll exercise later," start thinking, "If I exercise now, I'll accomplish more at work later because I'll have more energy and think more clearly." The idea that exercise comes before most aspects of daily living and enhances other aspects of life can lead to a change in thinking and help prioritize fitness.

—Aerobics and Fitness Association of America (AFAA)

Eventually, the goal is to exercise intensely for fifteen minutes, not four minutes. But we want to change habits—promote what's called cognitive restructuring—and build to fifteen minutes. But start small. *Four minutes*, just 240 seconds. That's less time than a block of commercials during your favorite TV show. That's shorter than most Top 40 songs. Less time than your average shower. Heck, most of us have been stuck at the light in a left-turn lane for longer than that. Four minutes. I mean, who doesn't have time for that?

Once you've convinced yourself that you can find four minutes for exercise, you're likely to ask another question.

What do I actually DO for those four minutes? And my answer is simple and can be reduced to three words: *It. Doesn't. Matter.*

Just as long as you move around at maximum intensity, doing vigorous exercise for four minutes a day. Whatever movements work for you. This is critical. This will spike your metabolism. Do that every day, because consistency is everything. But don't get hung up on the exercise. Just move like you mean it!

Such a simple instruction takes all the structure and complications out of the equation. Other exercise programs are too complex, especially for the obese, who often suffer from what I call low self-efficacy. They might have low self-confidence. They might have a fear of failure because they have tried everything and nothing has worked. They don't want a program that says, "On Monday you work your back and arm muscles, and on Thursday you switch to core and legs." Four minutes a day of vigorous exercise takes out all the programming.

You can shadowbox. You can do jumping jacks. You can do high knees. Whatever it is. You don't need to change clothes. You don't need equipment. You can do it inside or outside. You can do it in the morning, in the afternoon, in the evening, or in the dead of night. You have eliminated all the possible complications. Which means you have eliminated all the possible excuses.

After demystifying the exercises, I try to demystify the time. Again, four minutes isn't a big chunk of time. But it still has to become part of a routine. One strategy: build it into a routine that already exists. For drivers I might say, "You get in and out of your truck during each shift, right? It's part of your basic routine, right?"

Sure, they say, giving me a funny look.

"Well, every time you open the door to get into your truck, it's your choice. Do you want to drive with your metabolism on low, medium, or high? If you're already standing outside of your truck, why not move around for four minutes?"

Clients who aren't truck drivers also sometimes struggle with the time commitment. Not the four minutes, but, again, in building it into their routine. I ask them a simple question: Do you take a shower each morning?

Um, yeah.

So you're going to take off all your clothes, stand under running water for a few minutes, and wash your body with soap and shampoo?

Um, yeah.

And around the same time, before or after the shower, you're going to brush your teeth every morning?

Um, yeah. (Most say that, anyway. A surprisingly high number of people have the courage to admit to not brushing their teeth every morning. But that's probably a discussion best left for another time.)

Listen, I say. Those are two routines that you have already established. We're going to add a third routine that also goes to this goal of giving you an appearance you can be proud of. In the space between brushing and showering, or vice versa, you are going to add four minutes of vigorous exercise.

What do I mean by four minutes of vigorous exercise or high intensity? Basically that your breathing is hard and your heart rate is up. One easy way to tell your heart rate is up: you are breathing so hard that you have a difficult time getting a sentence out without stopping to catch your breath. (Another way to tell: buy a heart monitor and/or download a heart rate app.) You can achieve that in less than a minute. And you achieve this through literally hundreds of different exercises.

I will typically demonstrate to the class what four minutes of maximum effort means for me. This can include thirty to forty different exercises. Sometimes that means it's shadowboxing, standing in my bedroom and throwing straight punches and uppercuts. Other times it's doing squats. Other times it's lunges and lunge jumps. Other times it's push-ups—Spider-Man and dive bombers. Crunches, bicycle crunches. Russian twists. It's almost like I'm moving randomly from one to the next. But I go as hard as I can. And when I get tired of one, I move on to another. Hopefully, they watch me, see me huffing and puffing, and get the basic concept.

4-MINUTE MYTH BUSTER

"Longer workouts burn more fat."

WRONG!

I'm not knocking low-intensity workouts. Something is better than nothing. And, especially with older folks, or those who are obese or truly out of shape, starting with low-intensity workouts that don't stress the joints makes sense. But the notion that longer, lighter-intensity workouts burn more fat than brief, high-intensity workouts? That is just wrong. The truth is, when you exercise intensely, a higher proportion of the calories you burn comes from carbs. But because intense exercise burns so many more calories than light exercise does, you're still burning more total fat when you go hard. And more important, high-intensity exercise increases the size and number of your body's mitochondria—the "batteries" of your cells. It's the power of these mitochondria that determine how efficiently your fat-burning metabolic processes chug along. The intensity of the workout—not total calories burned during exercise—is the important measurement and the one that's going to determine how much fat you'll lose.

The average obese client isn't going to go through thirty different exercises. And they may not get through the entire four minutes. That's okay. Pick two, three, or four exercises. Maybe save the bicycle crunches for later, when you're in better shape. But jog in place. Move side to side. Do high knees. Can't do full push-ups? No problem. Do modified push-ups.

Can't do four minutes? No problem; most people can't when they start the program. All you can do is thirty seconds? Great. The important thing is that you're doing something, that you're in the game. Do thirty seconds a day that week. By the second week, your fitness will be a little better. Maybe then you're doing forty-five seconds. That next week, you're up to a minute, even 1:15. Trust me, you'll be up to four minutes before you know it.

When people ask to start slow and easy, I tell them that slow and easy isn't going to have a serious effect on your metabolism. You want to see rapid results? Go hard! You might feel silly at first, throwing punches into the air or running in place. That's understandable. But don't down-regulate or self-regulate. Do it like you mean it! It's much better to go at maximum effort for one minute than it is to be on cruise control for four minutes. You don't want to go so hard that you risk injury (more on this later in the book). But don't let self-consciousness or fear of feeling silly stop you from your goals.

4-MINUTE MYTH BUSTER

"You're not getting a good workout if you're not sweating."

WRONG!

Perspiration is our body's way of cooling itself. While it is an essential process, sweating depends on all sorts of factors, including room temperature. And it has very little to do with how many calories we might be burning or how hard we might be working out. That is, sweat is not an indicator of exertion. It's possible to have a high-intensity workout without doing a lot of sweating. It's possible to sweat a great deal without working out a great deal. (As anyone who's driven a truck in the summer with a busted air-conditioning system can attest.) Monitor your vital signs during a workout—starting with your heart rate—and you'll get a much more accurate gauge of your intensity.

And if you start off with the goal of losing weight rapidly, you're more likely to keep that weight off in the long run. A 2013 study in *The New England Journal of Medicine* found that when compared to people on a "slow and steady" weight-loss plan, people who pushed themselves to lose weight quickly were more likely to stick to their programs.

Testimonial: I DROPPED FIFTY POUNDS!

I'm down almost fifty pounds from my heaviest period. And I feel great. In a few weeks on this program, I had done what I couldn't accomplish in three-plus years of dieting on my own. —Travis Bacon, thirty-two

Testimonial: I LOST 100+ POUNDS!

I looked at [a photo of myself]—it was a full-body shot—and barely recognized myself. I'm about five foot eleven, and it turned out I weighed 340 pounds at the time. My body fat was something like 47 percent. Damn. I decided enough was enough and joined Siphiwe's program. When I finished the program, I was down to 228 pounds, more than one hundred pounds less! —James Peters, forty-one

Once you have developed a habit of doing four minutes of exercise, you've already succeeded in taking a huge step toward a lifetime of leanness. But now keep going. Increase your daily vigorous activity by a minute each week until you reach fifteen minutes. (This should take eleven weeks—not even three months—from when you hit the four-minute mark.) At that point it's all maintenance. You never have to go beyond fifteen minutes a day, every day. That's all you need to maintain for the rest of your life.

What I've noticed, though, is that once folks start down this path, they have a new lifestyle. They embrace the fitness lifestyle. And they want more. *Coach, what can you tell me about kettlebells? How do I get into using resistance bands? What's the best way to design a longer workout?*

4-MINUTE MYTH BUSTER

"People are overweight because they eat too much."

WRONG!

When I first starting working with truck drivers, I assumed that so many of them are overweight because of their own poor choices or their poor impulse control. I was convinced that overeating, combined with laziness, must be why two out of every three truck drivers are overweight or obese. But when I started my program and looked at the data I had, it turned out that wasn't the case at all. What I found: drivers—like most obese people—aren't gluttonous at all. Most of them are *undereating*, consuming fewer than three meals a day, more like 2.6 on average. A lot skipped breakfast, but some of them skipped lunch and/or dinner. Most people with a busy lifestyle do this, too. We eat twice a day and don't think much of it. (In fact, we probably assume it's good for us.)

And not only were the truckers I studied burning more calories than they were consuming, a lot of the time, their bodies were in full starvation mode. How could this be? Well, they weren't eating frequently enough, which means they weren't giving their metabolism any work to do during the day. Their metabolism had been turned down to the lowest level. They may overeat by the time they get to dinner, but the amount of food that they eat for dinner still wasn't enough to give them all the nutrition they need for the entire day. So they were actually *malnourished*. Nobody thinks of these big, tough, 300-pound truck drivers as being malnourished, but they are! And I've helped them turn their lives around. And if they can do it—if I can do it—then I know that you can do it, too.

A 4-MINUTE CALL TO ACTION

You just need to get up and move. For. Just. Four. Minutes. Each day. That's it. Four minutes, 240 seconds. If every American makes this a habit every single day, I believe we will win the War Against Obesity.

Why do I believe this? Because I am using this strategy within the most unhealthy occupation in America—long-haul truck driving—and it is working. And I have hard evidence to prove it. And if it can work for truck drivers who work and live in a unique environment with severe occupational obesity hazards, it can work for just about anyone.

It's real simple—do any movement or movements you can do, with maximum intensity, for four minutes.

In the trucking industry, 86 percent of America's drivers are overweight and 69 percent are obese. That's an *epidemic*. Imagine if 69 percent of your family were diseased. With such a crisis, you would think there would be a response by the trucking industry—an organized, coordinated response. But there isn't. There are a few programs here and there, but my program, Fitness Trucking's Driver Health and Fitness 13 Week Program, is the only system specifically designed for the industry. From 2012 to 2016, it was available only at one trucking company, Prime, Inc., in Springfield, Missouri, and it was a *voluntary* program.

So I realized that something needed to be done, and I set out on a campaign to revolutionize the world of long-haul truck driving by creating a culture of fitness within it. I had to design a program that would work for any driver, for people of all walks of life, fitness levels, and nutritional profiles. Something that was maximally effective and least disruptive. That program has become this book, *4-Minute Fit*.

Testimonial: I SAVED MY OWN LIFE!

The first time I went through Siphiwe's program, it was awesome. I ate six meals each day, three major ones and three snacks to keep the metabolism going. I did my exercise. Sometimes it was easy; other times I had to improvise. Sometimes it meant parking and running laps around my trailer. (Did you know thirty-two laps around a tractor trailer is a mile?) Then life happened, I had some personal setbacks, and got a little careless. It was the fall of 2015, I had turned fifty years old, and in three weeks I went from 245 to 220. It sounded like claims from the most outrageous diet. I knew, though, that something was wrong. Seriously wrong. I was diagnosed with DKA, diabetic ketoacidosis. It can lead to a diabetic coma. It's usually fatal. One of the first things I did was get back to Siphiwe's program. Now my blood sugar is heading down and so are the ketone levels in my urine. I'm back to eating better. I'm back to hating sodas and drinking water or unsweetened iced tea. I eat a lot of grilled chicken. I've given up canned food, like canned fruit that's been soaked in syrup. I'm back to exercising. I'm back to doing walks—doing those laps around the semi—and I'll be running soon.

I'm sticking with it this time. I'm committed, and no one can make me think any different. I'm 216 pounds and looking to get to 195 to 198. But I'm not out of the woods yet. And I probably will need to take the medication for the rest of my life.

What gets me is that all this was preventable. I'm here to tell you: this is no joke. This is your health. This is your body. And if you don't take it seriously—don't watch what you're putting in there; don't continue with the exercise and diet programs—you're going to be in trouble. That I am walking, talking today? It's a pure miracle, man. —Michael Phillips, truck driver, age fifty-two

I grew especially interested in the possibilities of 4-Minute Fit after reading *Opening the Energy Gates of Your Body: Qigong for Lifelong Health,* by Bruce Frantzis. The author explained that after the Chinese Cultural Revolution, the country's medical personnel—both Western and traditional—was dramatically reduced. More than half of the former practitioners fled the country; retreated underground; or, worse, had been killed. Meanwhile, the population doubled from 400 million to 800 million during the Mao era.

The government knew that it had a potential crisis on its hands. But in hopes of staving off a counterrevolution, the authorities took severe measures. And these measures worked. The national health problem stabilized until the quantity and quality of medical personnel was finally restored.

What did the government do? Frantzis explains: "They told the top tai chi teachers that they must design tai chi and qigong programs for the health of the general population. Many of these masters wanted to keep their secrets to themselves, so their families could retain their 'patents.' It has been said that the government insisted that they make their secrets public, or face the extermination of their families down to the last child or relative."

Here, according to Frantzis, is how it worked. When nonemergency patients visited the hospitals complaining about the chronic illnesses or discomfort caused by poor lifestyle or overwork, they were sent to a hospital administrator, who provided the patients with an ID card. The patients were then directed to nearby tai chi and qigong centers. If patients wished to qualify for another doctor's appointment or seek admittance to a hospital, they were required to have their card stamped every day for three months by a local tai chi or qigong instructor, certifying that the patient had shown up. The frequent tai chi and qigong sessions managed to stabilize the citizens' health, even in the face of poor sanitation and the starvation diet that most endured. During this brutal period from the mid 1950s on, it is estimated that between 100 million and 200 million Chinese people practiced tai chi or qigong daily.

Now, this got me thinking. Even during an almost unimaginably harsh period, China came up with a national fitness movement that accommodated 100 million to 200 million people. America has 169 million obese adults who are at the center of America's health care crisis. What is America's emergency response? What drastic measures has America taken to face the problem head-on?

The more I got to thinking about this, the more I realized there was no uniquely American movement to win the war against obesity. There was no Uncle Sam Wants You to . . . Exercise campaign. And that's when I realized that if my methods were working for obese truck drivers, they would work for all of America—if we could get all of America to do 4-Minute Fit!

3 Amazing Life Changes in Just 4 Minutes a Day

In 2010, without my knowing it, Robert Low—my boss at Prime Trucking and also the second vice chair of the Truckload Carriers Association—sat in a planning meeting. The discussion turned to the average life expectancy of long-haul truck drivers, just sixty-one to sixty-four years of age. For Robert, who had been in trucking most of his life, that statistic was beyond alarming. Why should the good men and women who drive his trucks, who sacrifice so much already, and are so indispensable to the American economy give up ten to fifteen years of their lives?

Somewhere in that meeting Robert made a deep personal decision to do whatever he could to improve driver health and fitness, not just at Prime, but throughout the industry. By the time I approached him in December 2011, with a business proposal to become the in-house fitness coach and devote my time to improving the health of the drivers in the fleet, he was already thinking along similar lines.

I knew the stats. And so did Robert. More than 90 percent of the employers in this country have some sort of corporate wellness program—a way to reduce health-care costs and also cut down on the absenteeism of workers who were spending more time than ever in doctors' offices and hospitals or at home feeling lousy. Having a corporate wellness plan could often save companies tens of thousands of dollars a year in insurance costs alone—and that's before factoring in lost work time, accidents, and other drains on the company's finances that could be caused by a fleet of unhealthy drivers.

But I also knew that most of these programs were fundamentally flawed. The *Harvard Business Review* found that only roughly 20 percent of the workers who had access to these kinds of programs ever took advantage of them, and even those workers who did use these programs rarely stuck with them. (One study found that half of the people who start a weight-loss program find a reason to give it up within the first six months.)

Having seen firsthand the obesity rate among truckers—and how this epidemic can impact a company's bottom line—my boss happily agreed to my business proposal. My mission was to revolutionize the world of long-haul truck driving by creating a culture of fitness within it. It was going to save money, and more important, it was going to save lives.

My goal was behavior change—giving drivers the knowledge, tools, confidence, and habits to lose pounds and then maintain a healthy weight for the rest of their careers. Not only would that save lives, but it would also prove that this program worked and would set my coworkers up for a lifetime of leanness and health.

But when I saw how *fast* the weight loss came, that was another sign that this was a special program that would be different from most company wellness plans, for one major reason: it was designed to help people lose a lot of weight, and fast. "Fast" matters: While "slow and steady" may have its advantages, studies show that the faster you can strip away fat, the more likely you are to stick to your weight-loss plan. In fact, you are more than five times as likely to succeed in your long-term weight-loss goals if you start out of the gate by dropping pounds rapidly, according to a 2013 study in the *International Journal of Behavioral Medicine*.

I determined that ninety days was just the right amount of time to get fast results while also teaching people a plan that they could master and stick to long after their initial ninety days were over. I implemented the Fitness Trucking 13-Week Basic Program, based on the 4-Minute Fit concept, and quickly drivers began losing weight. That was more than three years ago. Since then, thousands of drivers have been through the program and seen incredible weight loss and tremendous improvements in their health.

Most impressive, two out of every three drivers who start the program finish it to completion, a far higher completion rate than most other programs. And the average weight loss is 19.7 pounds. That's a big number, but remember, that's just *average*: Some drivers lost as much as thirty, forty, fifty, and even sixty pounds in thirteen weeks without skipping meals, and some who stuck with the program after the thirteen weeks went on to lose one hundred pounds or more.

In fact, the program was so successful that it outperformed both the weight-loss and fitness industries, including highly visible and heavily marketed programs such as Weight Watchers.

We found that 4-Minute Fit outperformed Weight Watchers in *three out of four categories*. This happened even though the 4-Minute Fit program used far fewer resources with a clientele that is more severely challenged and, remember, usually doesn't have access to kitchens or gyms.

FLATTER BELLY, LONGER LIFE

The Prime Trucking team was so successful in achieving weight-loss and fitness goals that drivers from other fleets began hearing about the program and then asking about it. So we branched out. Now drivers who don't work for Prime can use this system through Fitness Trucking, the consulting company we started. Thousands of drivers have lost weight, come off medications, even found boyfriends and girlfriends and gotten married.

Graduating from Yale? Winning swim meets? Traveling the world? Having all these adventures? None of it that compares to the feeling I get when people who have completed the program come up and thank me for turning their lives around. The truth is, they should be grateful to themselves. They're the ones who did it, who had the courage to start and the persistence to finish. But it's so gratifying to be part of their successes.

And that's why I decided to create this book, to expand my reach and bring this program from the interstates to Main Street. The techniques described in this book have helped countless truck drivers lose weight—a group without access to kitchens or home cooking; food storage issues; unable to get to the local farmer's market or to live on "health food"; restrained by their jobs from regularly getting to a gym; and with constantly changing schedules and interrupted sleep that create more stress than most of us ever have to cope with. If it can help them lose dramatic amounts of weight, then it can help you, too.

In fact, you should easily be able to match and even exceed the success that these drivers experienced, due to the simple fact that your life—as stress-filled as it may be—probably still offers you more fitness opportunities and better access to healthy food choices than the average truck driver has. But even if you spend eight to twelve hours a day behind the wheel, you can—and will!—achieve dramatic, life-altering improvements in every area of your life within just a few weeks (and in some cases, in just a few days). Here's what to expect in the next ninety days:

Your belly will get flatter, fast.

When our metabolism starts to dip, the first thing that happens is we begin to gain weight. But not just any weight: a lower metabolism sends fat directly to our abdomens.

And that's a key point: Just carrying around extra weight isn't necessarily the worst thing that can happen to your health. Where and how fat is distributed in your body are what makes all the difference. While the fat you collect around your chest, your butt, or your love handles is relatively harmless (it's called *subcutaneous fat*, meaning fat that collects just below the skin), the stuff that gathers inside your belly, pushing out your stomach and straining the fabric of your pants, is a very different animal entirely.

This belly fat, also called visceral fat, is a dangerous creature because, unlike other types of fat, it's metabolically active; it wraps itself around the internal organs (specifically the liver and pancreas) and uses that home base to generate a class of dangerous compounds called adipokines. (More about these in a moment.) In fact, according to a Mayo Clinic study of 650,000 adults, greater waist circumference means greater risk of death, at pretty much every turn.

Fortunately, belly fat is very sensitive to changes in metabolism; as soon as you begin to raise your metabolism, your body will begin to dispense with belly fat, and quickly. The dramatic weight loss you'll experience in the first ninety days will be primarily abdominal fat, and as a result, you'll see a drastic improvement in many other areas of your life, as well.

You'll slash your risk of diabetes.

Here's how dramatically belly fat impacts your diabetes risk: One study at Johns Hopkins University found that a man with a waist circumference of 40 inches is 12 times more likely to develop diabetes than a man with a waist of 34 inches or less. Another study in the *Journal of the American Medical Association* found that while people with high levels of belly fat had an increased risk of diabetes, those who store their fat in other parts of their bodies—that is, people who are heavier than they may wish but still have healthy metabolisms and little belly fat—don't have this risk.

But the belly fat epidemic is so out of control that by the time we reach the age of forty-five, about half of us have already developed elevated blood sugar levels that are often the precursor to full-blown diabetes, according to a 2015 study from the Harvard School of Public Health.

That's why increasing metabolism is the primary focus of this program. It's not about reducing calories, it's about turning on your metabolism to its highest level and then eating foods that keep the metabolism burning. In a trial that followed participants for more than eight years, researchers tracked two sets of people who had recently been diagnosed with type 2 diabetes. One set followed a "low-fat diet," while the second group ate plenty of lean proteins and healthy fats, the same kind of flexible, unrestrictive program you'll read about here. Those in the second group went significantly longer before needing diabetes medication, and more of them had their diabetes go into remission.

Your heart will get stronger and healthier.

In a study presented in fall 2013 to the American Heart Association, researchers reported following 972 obese people over eight years. They found that those who store most of their excess weight as subcutaneous fat were not at increased risk for heart disease, *no matter how much they weighed.* (In fact, storing fat in your hips, butt, and thighs may *lower* your risk of some health issues. A study in the journal *Cell Metabolism* in 2014 found that subcutaneous fat in your hips and thighs actually improves insulin sensitivity and reduces your risk of diabetes!) But patients with high levels of visceral fat were much more likely to develop heart disease, including heart attacks, strokes, heart failure, and atrial fibrillation (irregular heartbeat).

That's in part because visceral fat collects around your liver, the organ primarily responsible for producing and metabolizing cholesterol. As the liver becomes inflamed from all that surrounding fat, it begins to pump out more low-density lipoprotein (or LDL, the "bad" cholesterol that gums up your arteries). The result is like a jackknifed tractor-trailer in the middle of the highway; everything starts moving slowly or not at all. By attacking visceral fat where it lives (your belly, of course), 4-Minute Fit tamps down the troublemaker that's targeting your ticker.

And by the way, your liver takes a real beating from visceral fat as well. It's one of the reasons we'll be focused on reducing your carb intake: According to the Mayo Clinic, 1 in 10 cases of liver failure requiring a transplant now stems not from alcohol or drug use, but from abdominal fat. And as many as 10 percent of American children may already have suffered liver damage as a result of too much belly fat, according to federal surveys.

You'll get stronger, leaner, more well-toned muscles.

Earlier in this chapter, I mentioned *adipokines*. These compounds are produced by belly fat and then sent on their way to cause havoc throughout your body. Adipokines include such unsavory compounds as *resistin*, a hormone that damages your liver's ability to rid the blood of cholesterol; *interleukin-6*, a compound that contributes to arterial inflammation; *angiotensinogen*, a chemical that raises blood pressure; and *tumor necrosis factor*, which causes inflammatory diseases such as psoriasis and arthritis.

Among the many things adipokines do is to damage your muscles by decreasing their ability to store energy; that further hinders and reduces your body's ability to regulate blood sugar and increases your risk of diabetes. In a 2009 report by the Canadian government, researchers reported that gaining a few pounds can result in almost instant damage to your muscles: "[T]his development can be very rapid (i.e., within days), and precedes the increase in lipid uptake and accumulation that leads to insulin resistance." But 4-Minute Fit will restore your muscles to their leaner, healthier state and reverse the trend toward diabetes.

Your bones will get healthier, too.

And if you know about the importance of strong muscles, you know about the importance of strong bones, and how the two are interconnected. In a recent report out of Columbia University, researchers found that women with the most visceral fat had about 30 percent lower bone volume and greater bone stiffness and porosity than those women with the least amount of visceral fat.

You'll experience less pain and fewer injuries.

It's no surprise that weight gain is associated with back pain, knee pain, and just about every other kind of pain that comes with getting older. As we gain belly fat, the muscles of our midsections become stretched to accommodate the additional load. Because of this, they no longer have the strength to protect our lower backs, and general achiness—not to mention more severe injuries—ensue. Similarly, carrying around extra weight means more stress on our hips, knees, ankles, and feet—yet more places where aches and pains can develop. Some studies have even shown a link between obesity and carpal tunnel syndrome. Add that to the increased risk of arthritis and bone fractures, and it's clear that too much weight around your midsection is a recipe for physical discomfort.

You'll get smarter, and you brain will get bigger. Seriously. (Maybe.)

A few years ago, researchers performed a series of CT (computed tomography) scans on the abdomens of middle-aged women and men, to discover exactly how much visceral fat was hiding inside their bellies. Then they did CT scans on their brains. What they found was that the more belly fat people had, the smaller their brains.

Let me repeat that: *The bigger your belly gets, the smaller your brain gets*. At least that's what some research suggests. Why is this? It may be because the protein that metabolizes fat in the liver is the same protein found in the hippocampus, which is the memory and learning section of the brain. People who gain a lot of belly fat end up depleting this protein, making them 3.6 times more likely to suffer brain diseases such Alzheimer's later in life, according to researchers from Rush University Medical Center.

But if you lose belly fat, there's reason to believe that you'll regain your mental capacity. In a study at Georgia Regents University, researchers took obese and diabetic mice and put them on exercise programs to lose weight. They then tested the brain functions and memory capacity of the mice, and discovered that the animals actually performed better after their weight loss.

You'll find true happiness.

I've mentioned how so many of the people who've been helped by this program have gone on to find new loves, improve their existing relationships, and just become happier overall. But those feelings don't derive just from liking the way they look in the mirror more.

In a study published in the British journal *Age and Ageing*, researchers surveyed men between the ages of sixty and seventy-four on their physical health and their mental and emotional well-being. Then the researchers measured their testosterone levels and, using X-ray and MRI (magnetic resonance imaging) studies, measured their visceral and subcutaneous fat levels as well. What they discovered was that the greatest single factor impacting quality of life was visceral fat—the more belly fat these men had, the more likely they were to report unhappiness with their lives.

You'll make more money and save more money.

Weight gain costs us a lot of money—and not just because we need to buy new pants in bigger sizes. In fact, obese men spend an additional $6,500 more in annual health-care costs compared to men who maintain a healthy weight; women spend an additional $8,365 in potbelly penalties each year. In fact, by one estimate, obesity-related health care will cost Americans $190 billion this year alone.

Recently, Duke University took a look at 17,000 of its employees to see how their weight impacted their health-care costs. The results: well, let's just say that the more pounds you pack on, the greater the shadow you cast on your financial future. In fact, for each one unit uptick in body mass index (BMI)* above 19—which is the low end of healthy weight—a man's medical costs increased by 4 percent and his drug costs increased by 2 percent. Which says a lot, considering that the average American man's BMI is 26.6. (The average for American woman: 26.5.)

But the real cost of being overweight doesn't come in the form of prescription pills and diet products. It's not the money we spend on obesity; it's the money that obesity prevents us from making.

In a study in the *International Journal of Obesity*, researchers gave participants a series of résumés with small photos of the applicants attached. What did they learn? That the starting salary, leadership potential, and hiring decisions were all impacted negatively when the photo showed a person who was overweight. How do the researchers know that weight—and not their experience or general looks—was

---

* BMI is calculated from the weight of the individual divided by the square of the height. BMI calculators can be found on the Internet.

the deciding factor? Because they used the *same* individuals, before and after weight-loss surgery! And the impact seems to be greatest on women: One University of Florida study found that the thinnest women make a whopping $22,283 more a year than their overweight peers. For American women, gaining 25 pounds results in an average annual salary loss of $15,572.

You'll have (much) better sex.

Health and wealth are serious stuff, but I want to keep it real, and that means addressing what too much fat does to your sex drive. True, being overweight hardly disqualifies you from the game of romance; there are plenty of people of both genders who remain sexy and exciting and game in bed, regardless of how much they weigh. But dropping pounds, especially from the midsection, can do a lot for a woman's sex life. And it can do even more for a man's.

Sex is one of the most important and powerful sources of energy, inspiration, motivation, and happiness that exists in the universe. Men, women, old, young, straight, gay, across countries, cultures, and religions. This is universal. None of us would be here if it weren't for sex.

There is a line that is (mis)attributed to Freud: "Everything we do, we do to get laid." While that's an oversimplification, it gets at this point: A lot of what we do and how we act—directly or indirectly—is related to sex and these evolutionary forces. Part of wanting to go to work and earn income is to be more attractive to a potential mate. Same for why we put so much effort into appearance. We look at body type or we read the symmetry of someone's face, and we're often asking ourselves, consciously or unconsciously: *Is this person a potential mate? What are their genes?*

We spend a lot of time pursuing sex, thinking about sex. Sometimes it's for pleasure. Sometimes it's for reproductive purposes. But it's a significant part of life and, by extension, a significant part of leading a healthy life. Study after study will show that, overall, people who have a healthy sex life tend to have healthier lives and will generally live longer.

At an early age, most us are taught directly—or infer indirectly—that there's a relationship between our outward physical appearance and our sexual appeal. It's in the environment. Our culture reinforces it. This triggers what we call sexual attraction. So let's work on the assumption that we become more aroused when we see people who are fit rather than those who are unfit.

What does that mean for people who aren't fit?

I want to be clear: I have no data to suggest that obese people have less satisfying sex. But I've heard it anecdotally from drivers. And it makes sense. It means fewer people are likely to find them attractive. It's harder to find a mate when fewer people find you desirable. And if you don't feel good about your body, that can negatively impact your sex life. Sex is a most intimate act—maybe even *the* most intimate act—and it requires a degree of confidence and trust and even courage. If you're not confident about yourself, that has an impact on you sexually. Physiologically, it means that you are likely to have less sexual energy and tire easily. And—warning: I told you we're keeping it real here—the mechanics of sex become more challenging. We're talking about physics and geometry here. You have a hard time expressing yourself both in terms of projecting energy and doing things physically? Yeah, your sex life becomes less fulfilling.

I hear it all the time: as my drivers lose weight, it really begins to bolster their sex life. They have more energy in general, but also more energy for sex. As they lose the pounds and their clothes fit better—or they need new clothes entirely—their self-esteem goes up, and they feel better about themselves. As they have more confidence, they feel sexier. It's a virtuous cycle.

One of my favorite stories: A driver, Michael, went through my class and lost more than thirty pounds. It was the lightest he'd been in something like twenty years. Michael said, "Sip, listen, I gotta thank you, man. I met someone and we're engaged. And it was a direct result of just feeling better."

In the fall of 2013, I worked with Oscar and Joanne, a married couple who drive a truck on the road together—you'd be surprised at how many married couples do this—and they both wanted to lose weight. Joanne was around 200 pounds and lost more than 10 percent of her body weight with my program. Oscar was pushing 400 pounds and lost 53 pounds in thirteen weeks. He kept going and, with the help of a bariatric procedure, is now around 200 pounds, literally *half* his weight from when I first met him.

We're friends and, as you have probably figured out by now, I'm a direct sort of person, so I asked them straight up: "Guys, how is this weight loss affecting your sex life?"

Joanne's face lit up. "It's amazing! We used to have sex infrequently. Now it's more often and we go longer."

She explained that in the past, not only did Oscar used to get tired after a few minutes, but Joanne was afraid that her husband would fall asleep and roll over on her, causing physical injury. Imagine engaging in sex (and even trying to enjoy it) while your mind is worrying about your partner crushing you later that night!

They explained the cycle perfectly. As they got more fit and less overweight, they felt better about themselves. As they felt better about themselves, they felt happier and more energetic, which improved their sex lives. And the more that happened, the more incentive they felt they had to stay fit and healthy.

But there are other physiological issues to keep in mind. Consider this: as the abdominal fat pad grows, it swallows up everything around it. For guys, that means as we gain inches in our bellies, we lose inches elsewhere—inches we're not exactly eager to lose. So dropping pounds from your midsection can give you the illusion of having a bigger, more robust wingman.

But it's not just an illusion: high cholesterol, high blood sugar, and high blood pressure are all contributors to a lack of blood flow to the nether regions, a cause of sexual dysfunction for both men and women. And it can cause a dip in testosterone levels, which means a diminished sex drive and greater difficulty in maintaining a healthy sex life. But in a study in the *Journal of Sexual Medicine*, researchers found that losing just 5 to 10 percent of one's body weight over a two-month period increased both sex drive and erectile function in men.

So you could be smarter, richer, healthier, happier, sexier, and better looking. Or not. The choice is up to you.

4 The 4-Minute Exercise Solution

When you first saw the title of this book, your first reaction was probably "That's bulls**t." Get fit in just four minutes a day? Impossible.

But it's not, especially if that four minutes is daily, truly vigorous, and part of a fifteen-minute routine, and if you keep pushing your four minutes until you're able to do fifteen minutes of vigorous exercise a day.

BEGINNING YOUR METABOLISM-SPIKING EXERCISE PLAN

If you are severely overweight, it's possible that the closest you'll come to doing any exercise is watching a television commercial for some workout product. The thought of actually doing the exercise is intimidating in the extreme.

On the other hand, once you have made up your mind to take action, and you have built up your motivation, there is a tendency to overdo it—to do too much, too fast. Not so great! But it's easy for this to end up in extreme soreness and sometimes an injury. To prevent this and, just as important, to determine your exact fitness capacity, let's do this strategically, employing the minimum effective dosage for maximum results.

Remember, the point of 4-Minute Fit is NOT the extra calories you will burn during your four to fifteen minutes of exercise (that's an added benefit). Rather, it's *spiking your metabolism* in order to burn fat at an accelerated rate in both the short term and the long term. The following workout is designed to ease you into a fifteen-minute exercise routine, beginning with just four minutes of vigorous exercise. It is also designed to identify three exercises that you already feel comfortable doing and measure their metabolic effect.

STEP ONE: GET A HEART-RATE MONITOR.

To get the most benefits, I highly recommend using a heart-rate monitor of some kind. You can find them as cheap as $15 on some websites, or you can spend ten times that on a top-quality version. Either way, you need only a certain number of basic functions.

Most heart-rate devices will give you two numbers: your beats per minute (BPM) and your percentage of maximum heart rate (%Max). The goal is to get your %Max over 80 percent—the fat-burning zone—every single workout. By hitting that zone, you'll spike your metabolism and get your body burning more calories all day long, even if you're behind the wheel for hours at a time.

If you don't have a heart-rate monitor, you can use this formula:

► To find your maximum heart rate, subtract your age from 220. So, for a forty-five-year-old, his maximum beats per minute is 220 − 45 = 175 bpm.

► Now, to find your fat-burning zone, multiply your maximum heart rate by 0.8. So in this case, $175 \times 0.8 = 140$. That means that this person must get his heart rate over 140 bpm during each workout in order to have the effect of "spiking his metabolism."

When you're exercising in the fat-burning zone, your body will be burning high levels of calories. But again, the goal isn't to burn calories during the fifteen minutes you're moving; the goal is to burn calories during the other twenty-three hours and forty-five minutes of the day. When you spike your metabolism by hitting that fat-burning zone, and you keep feeding that furnace with regular doses of fuel every three hours, you put yourself into the twenty-four-hour metabolic burn zone.

STEP TWO: START STRATEGIC.

Most of us have seen *Rocky* or one of dozens of other sports movies in which a down-and-out figure throws himself into training, rebuilds his body, shakes off some form of adversity, and becomes a champion. And when we think of getting ourselves into shape, that's the model we have: Go big or go home. Feel the burn. Give 110 percent. No pain, no gain. Just do it.

Unfortunately, that's exactly the wrong way to approach weight loss, especially if you're significantly overweight or haven't exercised in a while. In fact, working out too hard or for too long will make it harder to lose weight.

That's because our weight is controlled not by how many calories we burn off during exercise, but by our metabolism. And our metabolisms reset themselves to adjust for long, tedious bouts of exercise.

Consider the studies of City University of New York researcher Herman Pontzer, who conducted research on an African tribe called the Hadza. Members of the tribe log long distances each day hunting and gathering, working extremely hard every day just to survive. So one would expect that they burn off an awful lot of calories on a daily basis.

But the CUNY researchers studied the metabolic function of the tribespeople, and discovered that in fact they burned no more calories during the day than the average sedentary American desk worker. Those findings inspired Pontzer to dive deeper into why. In a 2016 study in the journal *Cell*, Pontzer and his team measured the metabolic activity of 332 people from different countries, including the United States, Ghana, Jamaica, South Africa, and the Seychelles. They discovered that physical activity—i.e., exercise—accounts for only 7 percent to 9 percent of the difference in our daily calorie burn, no matter how active we are. And once we reach a certain level of physical activity, the other aspects of our metabolism—stuff like digestion, respiration, and so on—begin to slow down to conserve calories.

The good news, however, is that neither age nor gender seems to have any effect on our metabolism. The single most significant factor determining your total energy expenditure is *fat-free mass*. Unless you're planning on growing an extra pancreas, that means that adding muscle is the single best thing you can do to increase your daily calorie burn. So brief workouts that spike your metabolism and add lean muscle tissue do much more than long, slow, boring exercise sessions.

Here's how to get started creating your very own metabolism-spiking 15-minute workout.

Day 1: Write down your heart rate before you begin. Walk for fifteen minutes at the fastest pace you can handle and write down your heart rate every five minutes. That's it. Don't do any more.

Day 2: Write down your heart rate before you begin. This time, you are going to walk as fast as you can for four minutes and then pick any exercise that you can do—it could be push-ups, shadowboxing, squats, jumping jacks, et cetera. (See our complete list and description of the thirty-two best bodyweight exercises starting on page 69.) Let's call this chosen exercise (again, it could be any exercise you choose) "Exercise 1."

So you will walk for four minutes, then do Exercise 1 for 1 minute, and then write down your heart rate. Repeat this two more times for a total of fifteen minutes. Or, in other words, do three sets of walking fast for four minutes and one minute of Exercise 1 (at maximum intensity), measuring and recording your heart rate after each round of exercise. And that's it. Don't do any more.

Day 3: This is the same as Day 2, except you are going to pick a different exercise. Do three sets of walking fast for four minutes and one minute of Exercise 2 (at maximum intensity), measuring and recording your heart rate after each round of exercise. And that's it. Don't do any more.

Day 4: This is the same as Days 2 and 3, except you are going to pick a different exercise again. Do three sets of walking fast for four minutes and one minute of Exercise 3 (at maximum intensity), measuring and recording your heart rate after each round of exercise. And that's it. Don't do any more.

Days 5, 6, and 7: Do any combination of walking and Exercises 1, 2, and 3 that you want to do. You can vary the duration, the amount of rest, and the order in any way that you wish. And you can stick with one exercise for each workout or mix and match all three.

Again, the purpose of this is to establish the habit of doing fifteen minutes of exercise each day. For most people, learning a series of new exercises can be intimidating, so we eliminate that by allowing you to choose exercises you already feel comfortable doing. That lowers the learning curve. The important thing is that you do them with maximum effort for maximum intensity in order to spike your metabolism. *You want to use your heart-rate monitor to make sure you are working to over 80 percent of your max heart rate.* If you are, great! You don't have to learn anything new for the time being. All you have to do is those three exercises for the next few weeks. (If you are not effectively getting your heart rate up with those three exercises, then your combinations will require some modification in order to spike your metabolism. But that is good to know.)

Be honest and log it so you establish a baseline. Your goal is to try to get four minutes of vigorous exercise, but you're probably not there yet. That's fine. If you get only thirty seconds, that's fine. If you get halfway there and get to two minutes, great. But write that down. That's what you're going to do every day. That's all you do in Week 1.

Most people starting an exercise routine on their own are not going to take the time to learn the hardest exercises in the world and then start doing them. Rather, most people will start with the easiest exercises, ones they already know how to do. That's fine, as long as those easy exercises effectively spike your metabolism; if they don't, then you will end up wasting a lot of time without getting the results you want. So right off the bat you're going to know what exercises you like to do and how effective are they.

Finally, even if you feel like you can do more than this fifteen-minute routine, don't! My drivers make that mistake all the time. Some of them feel so good that they are finally outside, exercising, *doing something*, that the endorphins kick in and they feel great. Instead of stopping at fifteen minutes, they go on to walk for thirty or sixty minutes or even more. They don't feel the effect on their body at the time. And they won't feel it so much the next day either. But the second day—that's when something called delayed-onset muscle soreness (or DOMS, which we'll discuss later) kicks in. You will definitely feel extreme soreness if you have gone from doing no exercise whatsoever to doing too much too soon. I am not a big proponent of "killing" my clients on the first day or in the first week of starting an exercise program. I keep it simple and strategic—my own version of KISS!

WHAT TO EXPECT IN WEEK 2

In this first week, you're establishing your fitness base and working toward that four minutes of vigorous exercise, making this a part of your routine. In Week 2, you are going to push yourself to add some time to your vigorous exercise periods—but remember, don't go over fifteen minutes of total exercise! If you were able to go hard for a minute in the previous week, this week you're going to go for 1:10 or so. If you were able to go for 1:30 last week, this week you're going to push it up to 1:45. See the worksheet below for all your goals.

Fitness Goals Worksheet

1. Why are you reading this book?

2. What is your fitness goal(s)?

3. When do you want to achieve this goal?

4. What's motivating you?

5. What's really motivating you?

6. In answering questions 1 through 5, what/how do you feel? What emotions are you experiencing? (Note: Don't describe what you are *thinking*, instead identify what you are *feeling*.) It's important to identify your emotions. This is the source of the energy you will need to reach your goals.

    On a scale of 1 to 10, how satisfied are you with your:

    ▸ Weight?

    ▸ Health?

    ▸ The life you are living?

7. What is preventing you from answering 10 above?

8. What is most important to you?

9. Can you have/do number 8 above without your health?

10. What is your goal weight?

11. When do you want to reach that weight?

12. What has prevented you from reaching your goal weight?

13. Go back and look at your answers to questions 1 through 12. How much time and thought did you put into them? Did you give one-word answers? Did you write a complete sentence? Did you write a detailed paragraph? *How* you answered the questions says *more about* you and your motivation/readiness to change and succeed than *what* you answered.

14. Go back to the questions and dig a little deeper.

15. Why do you want to lose weight?

16. Whatever you answered to number 15, why is that?

17. Whatever you answered to number 16, why is that? (Note: This is how you dig deeper: you have to keep asking, Why?)

18. When will you start Week 1?

19. Which food-logging app are you going to use?

20. When will you schedule your fifteen minutes to get a minimum of four minutes of vigorous activity each day?

21. What will you say and what will you do when you don't feel like doing your workout, when you don't feel like logging your food, or you become aware that you are making excuses? (Note: if you don't have an answer for this, you are not properly prepared for success. Arm yourself ahead of time by having a plan for how you will behave.)

The key: we want to improve, but we're okay improving gradually. You've established the baseline, and now you just want to be sure you're getting a little bit better by this objective measures.

Here are three new exercises you can consider adding, which aren't overly challenging or unusual, but which can help you mix it up and spark your Week Two workout to get even stronger:

1. Knee Crushers

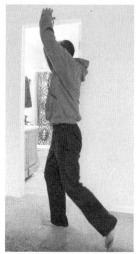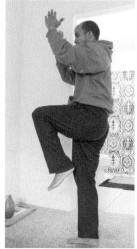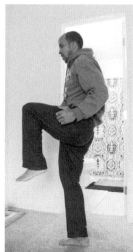

2. Shadowboxing

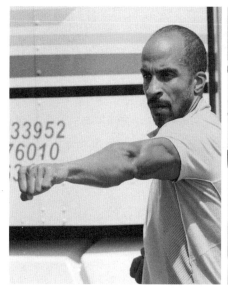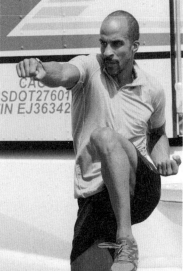

3. Squats

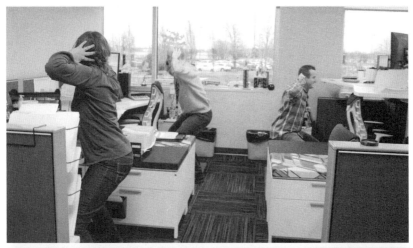

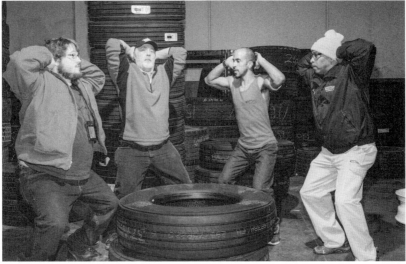

I'll say it again: we're just going for a little improvement each week. Not a lot, not great, massive, radical, life-altering changes. Just a little. But we want to do this for thirteen weeks. Not for two weeks, then backslide, then get back for a few more weeks.

Too often I see this: people start off and they are so motivated and so eager to change their lives—which is great—and they go like crazy at the beginning. But they can't sustain it, so they drop off. And when they drop off, their metabolism does, too. Then—whether it's guilt or disappointment or unhappiness with how they look or their energy level—they redouble their efforts and return to the program. Again, the spirit is to be applauded. *They want to get better.* Except now they want to make up for that lost time. And again, they can't sustain it and they tail off.

This is why the monitoring is so important. You don't want to do too much or too little. You want to do the right amount each week and you want to do it consistently. That's what will modulate all of this.

WHY LESS IS MORE

In this era of ultramarathons and Ironman competitions, fifteen minutes may seem like it couldn't be enough time to make a meaningful impact on your fitness. Hopefully, over the course of this book, I've convinced you otherwise. But if you're still a skeptic, try to look at it this way:

Imagine it's a hot day. You've been working hard, and you're thirsty. You drink a glass of lemonade, it's going to taste really good and satisfy you. Then you have a second glass that might be tasty, but probably a little less enjoyable than the first. By the time you get to a third or fourth glass, you might even be neutral. *I could take it or leave it.* Any glasses of lemonade after that, you're unsatisfied. In fact, you're probably officially sick of lemonade. Sometimes less is more and more is less.

This is called the *law of diminishing returns.* This holds true in all sorts of contexts. If you increase the output of a product, the quality is very likely going to go down. If you keep adding workers to a project, eventually they will get in one another's way and the enterprise will be less productive.

The law of diminishing returns is definitely in effect when it comes to exercise and fitness. In particular, it rears its head in "cardio training." The idea that you need to do cardio—generally considered to be exercise that will raise your heart rate—for twenty minutes or more? It is just plain wrong. Not only do you reach a diminishing return; you can get to a point where you risk *gaining* weight by doing too much cardio.

When you exercise, you are, of course, trying to burn fat for fuel. My body needs fuel to go on this jog or to ride this bike. Where does it get that fuel? One place is stored fat cells, where calories from carbs, proteins, and fats reside. Over time, though, the body will anticipate these long exercise sessions and it will respond to ensure that there's plenty of fat ready to be burned off. So, preparing for this, it will actually *conserve* stored body fat. In other words, because the body is designed to conserve fuel for the upcoming one-hour run or long cardio workout, it will basically stockpile fat in advance.

Long cardio can also undo the muscle mass you may be trying to add. Remember, muscle requires a lot of energy to maintain, so the more muscle you have, the greater your daily calorie burn. That's why resistance training for muscle growth is so important. In this chapter, I've provided you with a series of exercises that will spark your metabolism while preserving and even building more muscle.

In return, you just have to promise me one thing: no more than fifteen minutes of exercise a day, okay?

When you overdo it on the cardio, your body may choose to stop growing larger muscles—or even steal from them—because the demands on your body are for long, slow excursions, not big, powerful movements. So it decides that big muscles simply aren't necessary. So not only do you risk losing much of the muscle mass that you have been working so hard to gain, but this change has the effect of slowing down your metabolism in the process. There are several other reasons, too—some practical, some physiological—why I don't recommend extended cardio sessions. Consider:

- ▶ They can be boring. The less you enjoy an exercise, the less likely you are to do it. We all have different tastes, but I don't know too many people who enjoy those long runs on a treadmill or doing the same repetitive motion over and over. When I overhear people say things like "I forced myself to do X miles on the treadmill," I get skeptical about how long they can keep it up. You forced yourself? Hard to make a habit of something you don't enjoy.

- ▶ They can cause injury. The human body wasn't necessarily cut out for lengthy and repetitive exercise. It is the rare long-distance runner or endurance cyclist who hasn't had some form of injury from overexertion, whether it's joint pain or inflammation or shin splints or stress fractures or plantar fasciitis (a disorder that results in pain in the heel and bottom of the foot). Long, high-intensity exercise often brings injury with it. The problem isn't simply the discomfort or the fact that an injury to one part of the body often puts stress on other parts because of overcompensation. A real problem is that an injury can wreak havoc on your fitness goals and undo all the progress you've made.

- ▶ You are stressing your adrenal glands. Located just above the kidney, the adrenals produce hormones you cannot live without. Hormones have different functions but work together, at least when proportioned correctly. When we overdo exercise, we can trigger a fight-or-flight response, which cues the adrenal gland to produce more cortisol. This changes the ratio of hormones. When we do this repeatedly, the adrenal glands are taxed. Likewise, there are studies that conclude that long cardio workouts can have a negative impact on testosterone levels and, therefore, reproduction. One effect of a decrease in testosterone levels can be a decrease in muscle tissue. (As well as an increase in fat levels.) This ends in muscle wasting and can have the effect of slowing down your metabolism.

Bottom line: *less often means more*. A short but intense workout—where you're focused, you're getting your heart rate up, and hopefully you're having fun—is the way to go. The required time will be less. The triggering of hunger (and therefore temptation to cheat on your nutrition plan) will be less. The taxing of your body will be a lot less. And, at the end of the day, you'll get virtually the same benefits. In some cases, even more.

HOW TO MAKE A WORKOUT WORK BETTER

A vast body of research supports the idea that your environment affects the quality of your workout. People tend to have better workouts outdoors than indoors, for example.

There's also evidence that we have stronger workouts when someone else is present. Way back in the 1890s, a psychologist at Indiana University who was a cycling nut noticed that his fellow cyclists tended to post better times when they raced each other than when they raced the clock. He wanted to test this, so he devised one of the first lab experiments in social psychology. He concocted something he called the "competition machine" that resembled a rowing machine but with a wheel you turned with your hands.

First, the subjects exercised alone, seeing how many times they could crank the machine in a given period of time. Then the professor had them perform the same exercise in the presence of a peer. Consistently, the subjects were more effective when they were competing against someone else, not simply against a clock.

When working out, even if you're not competing with a partner, there are clear benefits to having someone else alongside you. There's more accountability. You tend to push each other—sometimes directly, other times subtly—so the intensity of the session increases. You tend to be less likely to stop short of a goal, for fear you might "lose face" with the other person.

The fact that someone is relying on you simply to show up will make you more likely to follow through on your commitment. If you bail and don't show up, you're not just letting yourself down; you're letting down someone else as well.

There is a downside, though. Remember: one of the organizing principles of 4-Minute Fit is simplicity, an assumption that it is maximally convenient. No set time. No equipment. You want to eliminate as many complications and potential excuses as possible. Well, when you chose to exercise with a partner, you're adding a layer of complexity. There are now logistical issues. When are you going meet up? Where are you going to meet up? What happens if someone is running late? What sort of exercise are we going to do? You might like burpees; your partner might prefer jumping jacks. There can be all sorts of other complications. *I want to work out with you, but I don't like working out with Sheila. Are you bringing her along?*

In the end, you have to make a decision: does the extra benefit I receive by having someone else present outweigh the added complexity that comes when another person is involved?

FAQ: Should men and women exercise differently?

No! I've talked to countless women who want to improve their fitness but are reluctant to lift weights because they're afraid of adding bulk and looking too masculine. And how many times do you go the gym and see men working exclusively on their arms and chests, neglecting their legs or their cardiovascular fitness?

Male and female bodies are far more alike than they are different. And we lose or gain muscle or fat in much the same way. But our bodies also have a natural, healthy shape, either masculine or feminine, and exercise is the way to attain that shape. It's no more possible for a woman to become "bulky" or overly muscular through regular exercise than it is for a man to develop an hourglass figure. That sort of transformation takes years of intense workouts, highly calibrated nutritional supplements, and often the use of controlled substances. Under normal conditions, male and female muscles and metabolisms work the same way, but the workouts yield different results. If you and your spouse or partner want to lose weight and get healthier, there's no reason you can't share a routine.

TO STRETCH OR NOT TO STRETCH?

If "stretching" were a stock in a company traded on Wall Street, you might want to sell it.

There was a time, not long ago, when stretching was considered essential to exercise. You would go to a gym and you would see as many people stretching as you would see people actually exercising.

The thinking was: (a) it warmed up the muscles, and (b) it increased flexibility, and this greater range of motion would prevent injury.

Since then, research has come out suggesting that maybe stretching before exercise isn't as important as we thought it was. It doesn't necessarily reduce muscle soreness or prevent injury. In fact, most informed trainers nowadays will say that it's best to stretch *after* exercising, when the muscles are warm. This will prevent injury, help rest muscle fibers, and flush out waste built up in the muscles as a result of exercising. This will make you a little less sore the next day, which will increase your ability to perform. Stretching before exercise, when the muscles are not warmed up, can lead to injury and can actually weaken the muscle just before you start exercising. So you definitely don't want to do that.

I think it's a personal choice, something optional and not mandatory. Some people feel their bodies need it to get the blood flow going and move better. Others don't feel that benefit. Some people use it for a period of relaxation before or after a workout, almost more mental stretching than muscle stretching. Other people would prefer to get in and out.

Me? I do the same thirteen-minute yoga stretching routine every morning, as soon as I wake up. That's how important stretching is to me. I don't feel right if I don't stretch before I start my day. I have learned from those who are stretching experts that stress is stored in ligaments and tendons. That is one of the reasons yoga relieves stress—it stretches the ligaments and tendons, along with the muscle. Then there's the entire mind-body connection that one can engage through stretching, moving, and breathing. So just in terms of general well-being, stretching is something I believe is so important that I make sure I do it before I do anything else each day. But that's just me.

That said, for those of us with sedentary jobs, there is one part of the body that needs stretching regularly: *the hip flexors*. The hip flexors are two thick bands of muscle that run alongside your pelvis, connecting your spine to your upper thighs; whenever you lift a knee, you're using your hip flexors. But when you sit passively all day, with your knees bent, the hip flexors tighten and shorten, causing bad posture, improper force loading on joints, and ankle, knee, hip, lower back, neck, and shoulder injuries. Stretching regularly each day can prevent this.

TIGHT HIP FLEXORS

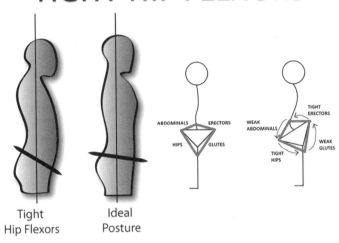

Tight
Hip Flexors

Ideal
Posture

Here's a simple stretch for that part of the body:

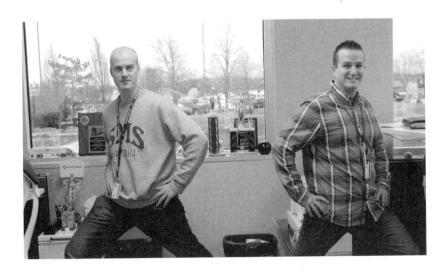

NO PAIN, PLENTY OF GAIN

Remember the John Mellencamp song "Hurts So Good"? It can apply to exercise, too. Especially in the beginning—and especially when we're just starting to begin a fitness regimen or are undertaking unfamiliar activity—one by-product of exercise is soreness. You bend down to tie your shoe, and you feel it in the back of your legs. You get up from your desk, and you feel it in your back. Yes, you even rise from the toilet and you feel it in your glutes.

"It" is delayed onset muscle soreness, or DOMS, as it's more commonly known. DOMS usually rears its head (or its arm or back) several hours after your workout. And it peaks at around the forty-eight-hour mark. While DOMS has been around since humans first started moving their body parts, it was long misunderstood. For decades, trainers and even some doctors attributed DOMS to lactic acid buildup. That's since been disproven. Now DOMS is believed to be caused by microscopic tears in the muscle. Those tears lead to muscle growth, so DOMS can indeed be a sign that you're getting stronger.

DOMS isn't pleasant. But it's not agony, either. And while it's irritating, it's also strangely satisfying. We've all heard the saying *No pain, no gain*. With DOMS we often tell ourselves, "Well, it must have been a good workout, if I'm feeling it this morning." But while a little stiffness is nothing to be concerned about, experiencing intense muscle soreness on a regular basis will prevent you from hitting your fitness goals.

When you work out vigorously on a Saturday and are still sore on Monday, how do you think Monday's workout is going to go? Not well.

There are four simple ways to prevent DOMS and ensure that your workouts, and your body, are operating at maximum efficiency.

PAIN SAVER 1: Start slow. The first step to preventing DOMS is not to do too much too fast. I often tell obese clients to do nothing more than walk for fifteen minutes on Day 1. I can't tell you how many times they walk for an hour. *Hey, that wasn't so bad; I knew I could do more than a measly fifteen minutes.* But then complain a day later that their legs are stiff and sore.

"Why did you walk for more than fifteen minutes?" I ask.

"Because I felt great and knew that I could keep going after I hit the fifteen-minute mark."

"You're right," I'll respond. "You *could* walk for more. But you hadn't walked for an hour in years. And now your body is telling you that it was too much. Don't do more than what the protocol says."

PAIN SAVER 2: Always eat after the workout. When you exercise at a high intensity—even if it's just for a minute—you're depleting your body of nutrients. If, right after you exercise, you give back to the body some of the nutrients you depleted, you help to speed along the repair work. If you don't eat anything, your body will start to try to repair itself and won't have the resources. As a result, the microscopic tears in your muscle tissue caused by exercise—the very things that help your muscles get stronger and get your metabolism revving—won't get repaired as efficiently. That means not only that you'll feel the impact of those tears the next day, but also that you won't build strength and endurance as quickly as you could.

PAIN SAVER 3: Stretch after your workout. By stretching *after* the workout, when the muscles are warm, you reset the fibers.

You trigger the removal of the waste products that build up when you exercise. You also stimulate blood flow, which helps to deliver more nutrients to your muscles, speeding recovery.

PAIN SAVER 4: Roll it. Finally, for the type A personalities in particular, I am a big fan of foam rolling. This is like an extra-credit tip. It's adding time to your workout program. (And a little added expense, too.) And it's a little hard-core. But it works. Foam rolling is a self-massage technique that stretches muscle fibers and connective tissue otherwise missed by traditional stretching. It also helps to soften the fascia, the thin lining of connective tissue that covers the muscles. (Think of the transparent lining you often find on raw chicken breasts—that's the fascia.)

But let's say that one day your exuberance takes over, you do more during a workout than you should, and you don't have time to stretch afterward. It happens. You wake up the next day feeling like your muscles are in revolt. Now what do you do? Well, a cold bath helps. Studies have shown that a five-minute ice bath will reduce swelling by 20 percent. But that's for severe cases; for most of us, even a few minutes in a cold shower will help reduce swelling and inflammation.

Finally, there are Tylenol and other analgesics. In many cases, the majority of the pain you feel isn't from the damaged muscle itself, but from surrounding muscles tightening up in an effort to prevent further damage to the injured area. Muscles sometimes behave like the mafia; they close ranks and protect their own. You can help break this cycle with analgesics, which both restrict blood flow to the injury (reducing inflammation and soreness) and decrease the perception of pain by reducing the flow of pain signals from the brain.

Bottom line: Soreness may "hurt so good." But you don't need discomfort to prove to yourself that you had a strong and productive workout.

THE 32 MULTI-MUSCULAR EXERCISES OF 4-MINUTE FIT

- ▶ *The Journal of Physiology,* 2010: "*A practical model of low-volume high-intensity interval training induces mitochondrial biogenesis in human skeletal muscle.*"

- ▶ *Science Daily,* March 2010, "*High-Intensity Interval Training Is Time Efficient and Effective*": "*A study at Laval University in Quebec, Canada, found that HIIT cardio helped trainees* lose 9 times more fat *than those who trained the traditional way.*"

- ▶ *Men's Journal*, August 2013: "*High-intensity interval training is one of the best ways to get in shape. It's also brutally efficient . . . Go hard. Rest briefly. Go hard again. That's the essence of high-intensity interval training . . . Now, after decades of research, exercise physiologists are finally explaining the outsize health and fitness impact of these ferocious little workouts—vastly greater, for every minute invested, than longer, slower efforts . . . 'You can get a lot of fitness benefit with these very short-burst workouts,' says Steven T. Devor, associate professor of kinesiology at the Ohio State University. Same for the health benefits: 'It is becoming quite clear that you get lower body fat, lower risk for disease, lower LDL cholesterol and higher HDL, and lower blood pressure,' he says.*"

- ▶ *Muscle & Fitness,* October 2014: "*High-intensity interval training is the future of fat burning . . . One study at a time*

HIIT knocked steady state cardio off its long-held throne, be-coming the most relied-upon method for burning unwanted body fat in gyms everywhere . . . This type of training is not only being used by athletes to improve conditioning but also by trainers and their clients as one of the best methods for fat loss and conditioning. With our busy lifestyles, who has time to do 40–60 minutes of aerobic training? The scientific data now show that less is better when it comes to fat loss—you just have to know how to do it right." (Justin Grinnell, CSCS, per-formance coach and owner of State of Fitness in Michigan.)

Each of these exercises will call into play a number of muscle groups. The more muscle groups you call upon, the more your body is triggered to create ATP, and the greater your metabolism boost will be. Select any of these to work into your daily routine.

Dip

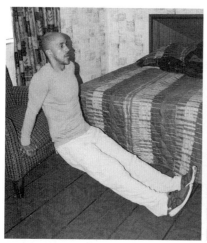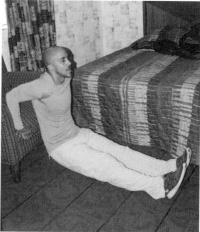

Sit on the floor with your back against a low bench and your legs straight. Reach your hands back and rest your palms on top of the bench so that the weight of your upper body is supported by your arms and shoulders, and your elbows are bent. Now straighten your elbows and push yourself up until your arms are straight and your full body weight is supported by your palms and the heels of your feet. Slowly bend your elbows and lower your body toward the floor, stopping before your lower body touches the floor. Pause, then push yourself back up again.

Squat

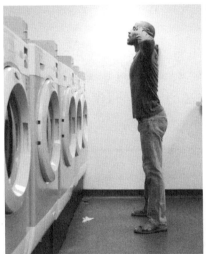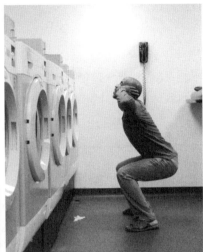

Stand with your feet shoulder width apart. Reach both arms out in front of you, palms down. Or place your palms on the sides of your head. Slowly bend your knees and lower your buttocks as though you were sitting down in a chair. When your thighs are parallel to the floor, pause, then push up with your feet and return to the starting position.

Lunge

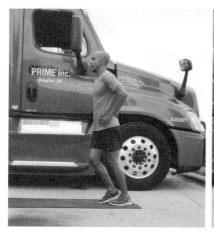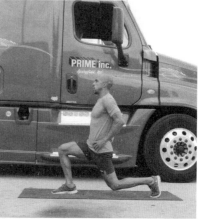

Stand with your feet shoulder width apart. Step forward with your right leg, bending your right knee until your right thigh is parallel to the floor. Your left knee should be bent and almost touching the floor. Push up with your right foot and return to the starting position. Repeat with the left leg.

Push-up

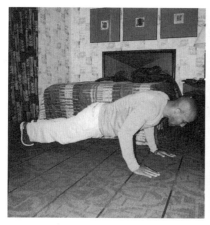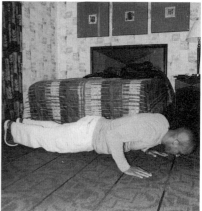

Lie facedown on the floor with your hands at your sides at chest level, palms against the floor. Keeping your back straight, straighten your arms to push your body upward until your arms are fully extended and your weight is balanced on your palms and toes. Try to keep your back rigid throughout the movement. Lower back down to the starting position.

Squat Jump

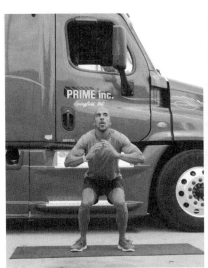 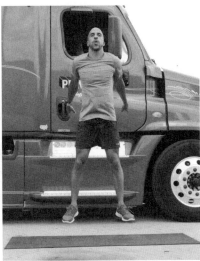

Stand with your feet shoulder width apart. Reach both arms out in front of you, palms down. Slowly bend your knees and lower your buttocks as though you were sitting down in a chair. Now swing your arms upward as you push off with your feet and propel yourself upward into the air. As you land, extend your arms and return to the squatting position. Repeat.

Pistol Squat

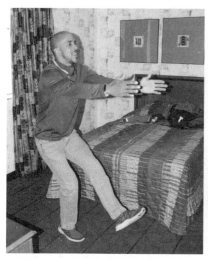 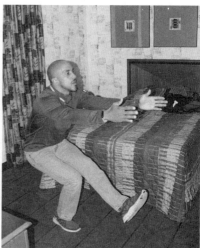

Stand with your feet shoulder width apart. Reach both arms out in front of you, palms facing each other. Extend your left leg out in front of you, keeping your knee straight and your weight balanced on your right leg. Maintaining your balance, slowly bend your right leg until your right thigh is parallel to the ground, keeping your arms and left leg extended out in front of you. Pause, then push up with your right leg and return to the standing position. Repeat with your right leg extended and your weight balanced on your left leg.

Lunge Jump

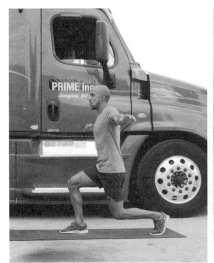
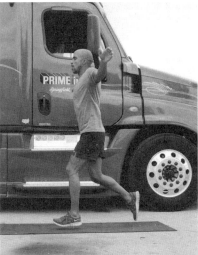
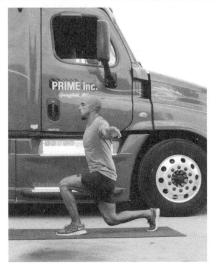

Stand with your feet shoulder width apart. Jump up into the air and extend your right leg, so you land with your right knee in front of you and your right thigh parallel to the floor. Your left knee should be bent and almost touching the floor. Push up with your right foot and return to the starting position. Repeat with the left leg.

Jumping Jack

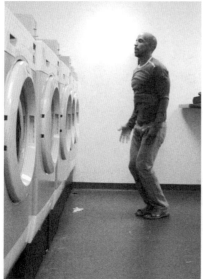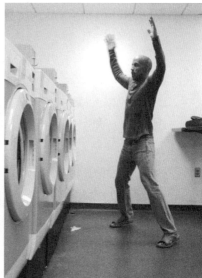

Stand with your feet shoulder width apart and your hands at your sides. Jump into the air, spreading your feet and extending your arms into the air, touching your hands together over your head. Land with your hands together and your feet spread wide. Immediately jump back into the air and return your hands and feet to the starting position as you land. Repeat.

Shadowboxing

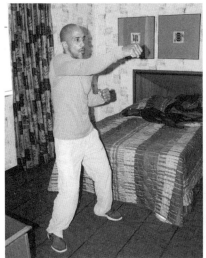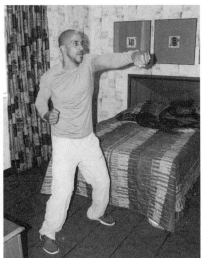

Shuffle your feet forward, backward, and side to side as you throw punches at an imaginary opponent. Use combinations of punches in rapid succession; the faster the combinations, the more effective the workout.

Running in Place

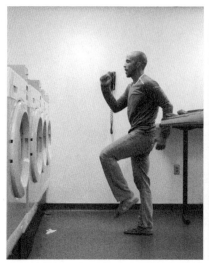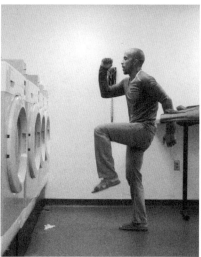

Jog in place using both your arms and legs. The higher and more vigorously you lift your arms and legs, the more effective the workout.

Spider-Man Push-up

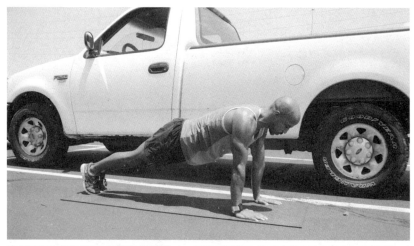

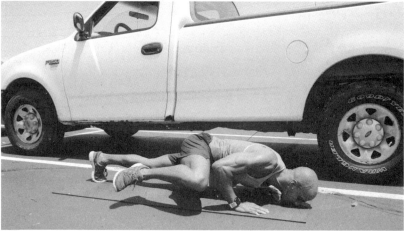

Start in a push-up position. As you bend your arms to lower your chest toward the ground, bring your right knee up to meet your right elbow. Then press up and return to the push-up position. Repeat, bringing the left knee to meet the left elbow.

Single-Leg Ice Skaters

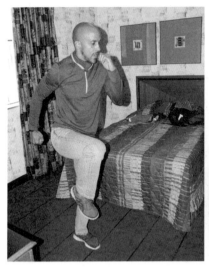 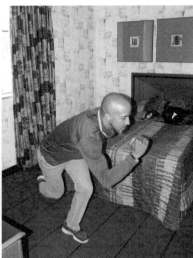

Stand with your feet shoulder width apart. Jump to the left and land on your left leg, with a slight bend in your knee; keep your right foot off the ground. Now jump to the right, landing on your right foot and keeping your left foot off the ground. Repeat.

Dive-bomber Push-ups

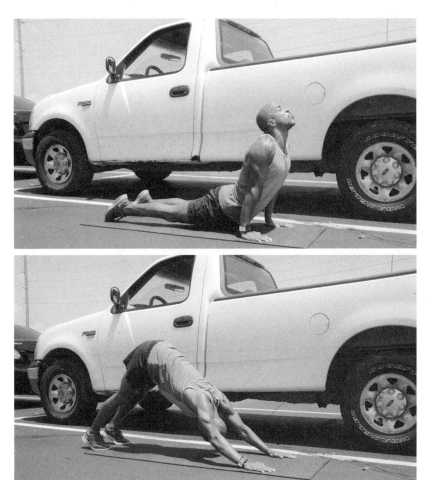

Lie facedown on the floor with your hands at your sides at chest level, palms against the floor. Push your hips up as high as possible so that you resemble an inverted *V*. Now lower your hips, keeping your legs straight and bending your arms so that your chest is lowered almost to the floor. Push back up with your arms until you have returned to the inverted *V* position.

MMA-Style Knee Raises

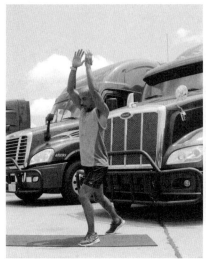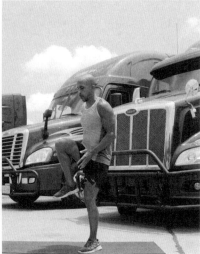

Stand with your feet shoulder width apart. Take a step backward with your right leg and bend your left knee. Raise both hands above your head. While bringing your right leg up and bending the right knee until your thigh is parallel to the floor, bring both hands down to meet the right knee. Now extend both arms over your head again as you return the right leg back to the starting position. Do several repetitions and then switch to the left leg.

Shadowboxing with Kicks

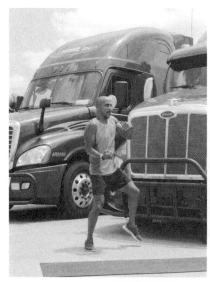 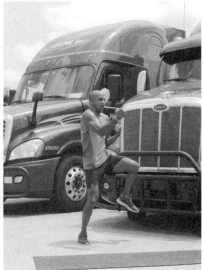

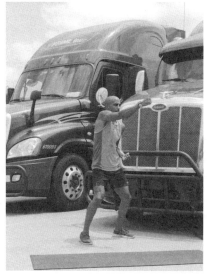

Shuffle your feet forward, backward, and side to side as you throw punches and kicks at an imaginary opponent. Use combinations of punches and kicks in rapid succession; the faster the combinations, the more effective the workout.

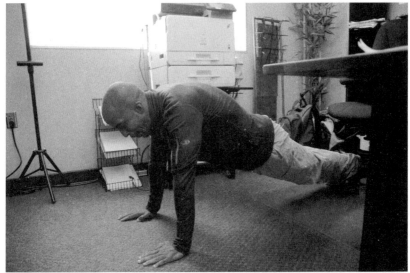

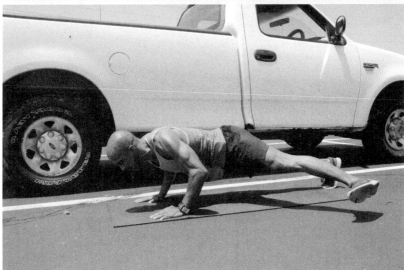

Lie facedown on the floor with your hands at your sides at chest level, palms against the floor. Keeping your back straight, straighten your arms to push your body upwards until your arms are fully extended and your weight is balanced on your palms and toes. Try to keep your back rigid throughout the movement. As you reach the top of the movement, lift your left foot off the ground and extend your left leg as high up as you can. Return the left leg to the floor and then lower your body back down to the starting position. Repeat using the right leg.

Hops

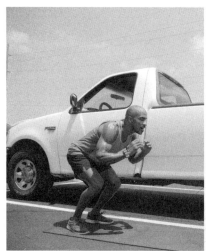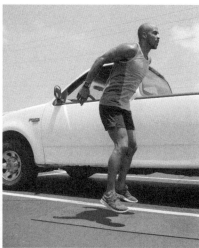

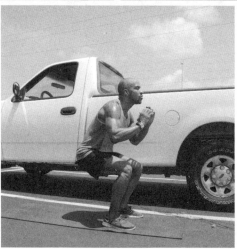

Stand with your feet shoulder width apart and your hands at your sides. Bend your knees and crouch down as you swing your hands behind you. Now swing your hands forward as you jump forward explosively and land on both feet. Crouch down and jump to the left explosively, landing on both feet. Crouch down and jump backward explosively, landing on both feet. Crouch down and jump to the right explosively, landing on both feet. You should wind up at approximately the same point you started from.

Planks

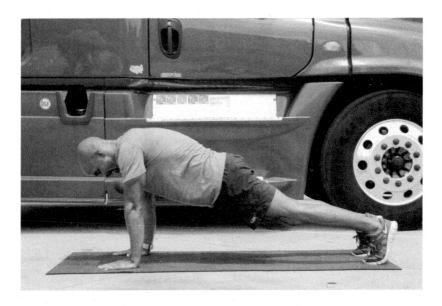

Lie facedown on the floor with your feet together, your elbows bent, and your forearms or palms against the floor. Keeping your back straight, brace your abdominal muscles and push your body up so that your weight is resting on your toes and your forearms or palms. Hold this position for as long as you can, working up to thirty to sixty seconds. Repeat.

Burpees

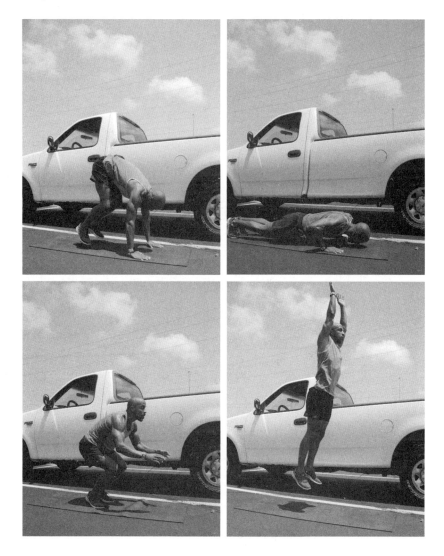

Stand with your feet shoulder width apart and your hands at your sides.

Jump down and place your hands on the floor, shoulder width apart, with your weight resting on your hands and toes and your knees bent, feet below your hips.

Pushing off with your hands, extend your legs backward until your legs are straight and your weight is resting on your hands and toes.

Bend your elbows and lower your chest until it nearly touches the floor, then straighten your arms and push back up.

Bend your knees and jump your feet back under your hips.

Jump into the air, spreading your feet and extending your arms into the air, touching your hands together over your head. Land with your hands together and your feet spread wide.

Immediately jump back into the air and return your hands and feet to the starting position as you land. Repeat.

Step-ups

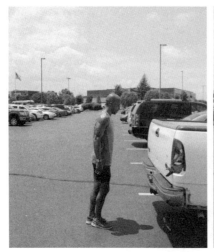 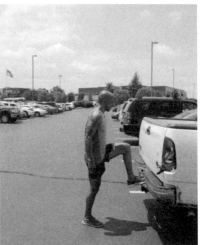

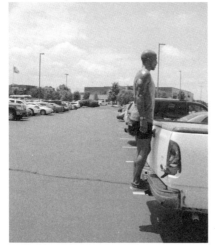

Stand in front of a bench or stair. Bend your left leg and place your left foot on the bench. Pushing off with your left foot, straighten your left knee until you're balanced over the bench on your left foot. Keep your right foot behind you so your weight remains on your left leg at all times. Now bend your left leg and return your right foot to the floor. Step your left foot down off the bench and return your left foot to the floor. Repeat the motion with your right leg.

Crunches

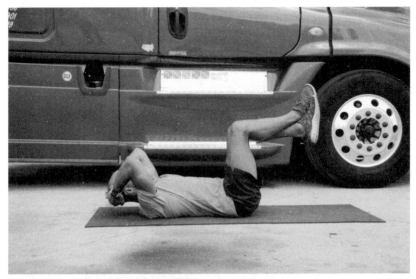

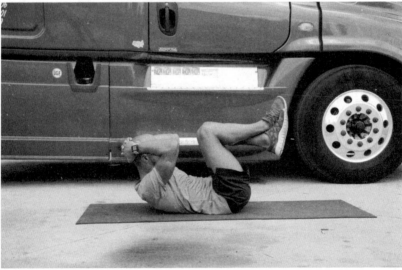

Lie on the floor with your knees bent, feet raised. Lace your fingers behind your head. Contract your abdominal muscles as you slowly curl upward, lifting your shoulders and upper back off the floor. Pause for a moment, then slowly lower your upper back and shoulders to the floor. Repeat.

Bird Dogs

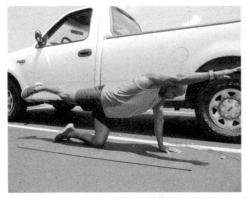 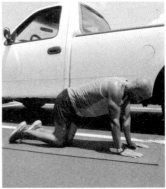

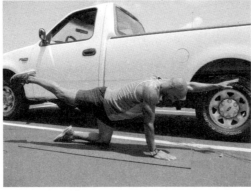

Get on the floor on your hands and knees. Extend your left arm out in front of you as far as you can. Simultaneously extend your right leg out behind you as far as you can. Return to the starting position, then repeat using your right arm and your left leg.

Side Planks

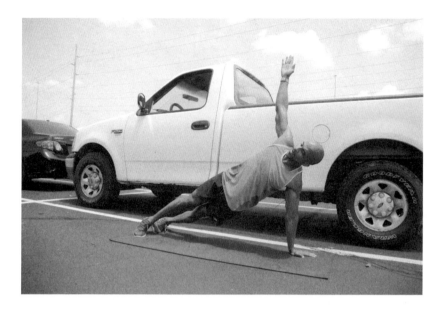

Lie on the floor on your left side with your feet together and your left elbow bent, left palm resting on the floor. Brace your abdominals, then lift your hips upward so that your weight is resting on your left hand and left foot. Keep your hips and torso straight; don't let them sag toward the floor. Hold this position for as long as you can, working up to thirty to sixty seconds. Lower back to the floor, then repeat on the right side.

Bench Jumps

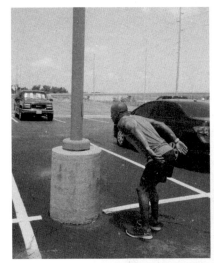 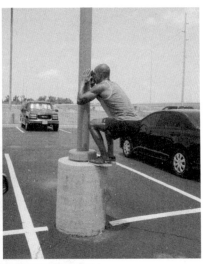

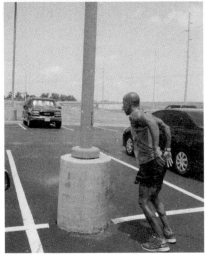

Stand in front of a low bench or step with your feet shoulder width apart. Bend your knees and extend your arms behind your back. Now extend your knees and swing your arms forward as you jump up onto the bench with both feet. Pause for a moment, and then carefully step back down to the starting position. Repeat.

Russian Twists

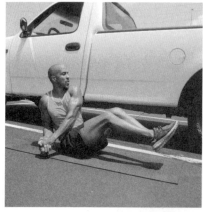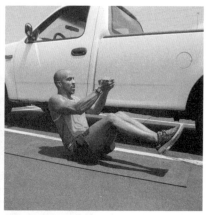

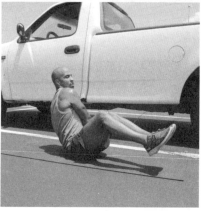

Sit on the floor with your feet extended out in front of you, legs slightly bent. Extend both arms straight out in front of you. Lift your feet off the floor and balance your weight on your buttocks. Now brace your abdominals and twist your upper body to the left until your arms are extended out to the left. Twist back to center, then twist to the right until your arms are extended out to the right. Repeat.

Bicycle Crunches

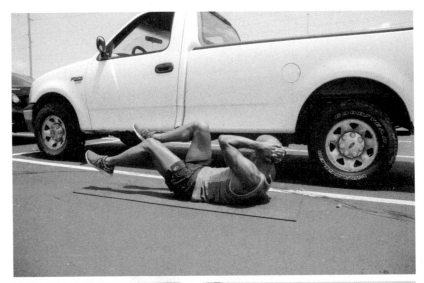

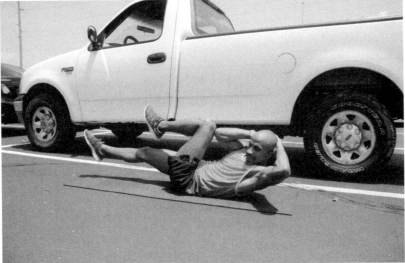

Lie on the floor with your knees bent and your thighs perpendicular to the floor. Place your hands at the sides of your head so your elbows are bent and your fingertips are just lightly touching the sides of your ears. Bend your legs so you curl your upper body upward to lift your shoulders and upper back off the floor; simultaneously, twist your upper body to the left. As you curl up, bring your left knee toward your head and try to touch your right elbow to your left knee. Return to the starting position, then immediately repeat to the other side, trying to touch your left elbow to your right knee.

Mountain Climbers

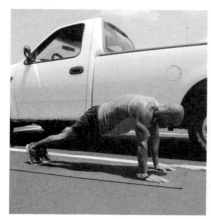
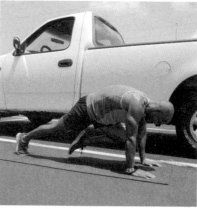
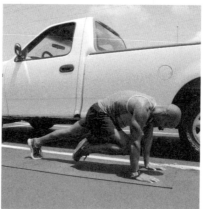

Get on the floor on your hands and feet, with your knees slightly bent and your feet extended behind you. Quickly drive your right knee toward your chest, bringing your right foot underneath your torso, then lift your right foot and bring it back to the starting position. Repeat with the left foot. Repeat the sequence as rapidly as you can.

In-and-Out Crunches

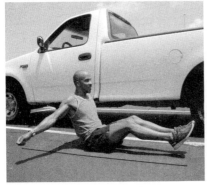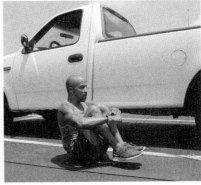

Lie on the floor on your back with your feet extended and your arms straight, hands at your sides. Lift your upper back and shoulders off the ground, and simultaneously lift your feet off the ground about an inch or so, so your body weight is resting on your lower back and buttocks. This is the starting position. Now curl your body upward as you bend your knees and bring them toward your chest. Reach your arms out so they extend to touch the sides of your calves. Straighten your legs and lower your upper body to return to the starting position, then repeat.

Hand-to-Toe Crunches

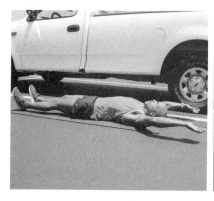 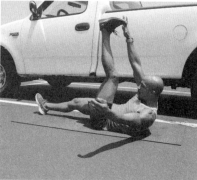

Lie on the floor on your back with your feet extended and your arms straight, hands above your head. Lift your left leg until it is pointing toward the ceiling, perpendicular to the ground. Extend your right arm upward toward your foot. Now curl your shoulders and upper back off the floor, trying to touch your hand to your foot. When you've gone as far as you can, pause for a moment, then lower your upper body back down and repeat with the other leg.

Side Planks with Leg Raises

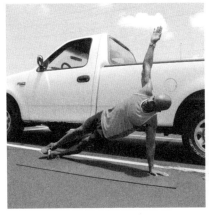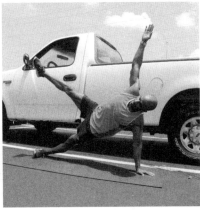

Lie on the floor on your left side with your feet together and your left elbow bent, left forearm resting on the floor. Brace your abdominals, then lift your hips upward so that your weight is resting on your left hand and left foot. Keep your hips and torso straight; don't let them sag toward the floor. Now lift your right leg toward the ceiling, hold for a moment, and lower it back down. Repeat this motion while holding the position for as long as you can, working up to thirty to sixty seconds. Lower back to the floor, then repeat on the right side, performing the extensions with your left leg.

Side Planks with Hip Thrusts

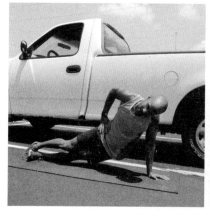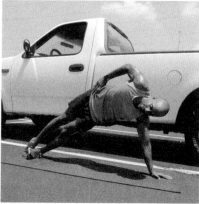

Lie on the floor on your left side with your feet together and your left elbow bent, left hand resting on the floor. Bend your knees slightly so your feet are just behind your buttocks. Brace your abdominals, then lift your hips upward so that your weight is resting on your left hand and left foot. As you lift, keep your feet together, but spread your knees apart, creating an "open clamshell" position. Bring your knees back together as you lower your left hip to the ground. Repeat 10 times, then change position so that you are lying on your right side, and repeat the motion with your weight rested on your right hand and right foot.

Side-to-Side Toe Touch Jumps

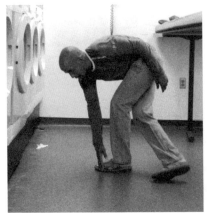
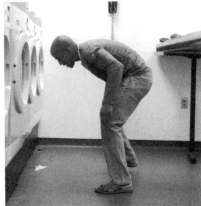
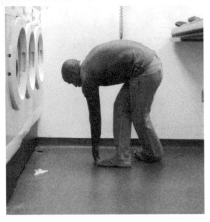

Stand with your feet shoulder width apart. Jump to the left and land on your left leg, with a slight bend in your knee and touch the outside of your left foot with your right hand; keep your right foot off the ground. Now jump to the right, landing on your right foot and touching your right foot with your left hand, while keeping your left foot off the ground. Repeat.

5 How We Got So Fat–and How to Drop the Weight, Fast

What do Hollywood, the boating industry, and your local lingerie store all have in common? They've all had to change their businesses to accommodate our increasing girth.

Movie theaters now spend nearly one third more on their building space than they did in the 1990s. Why? It's thanks to the need to increase the size of theater seats to accommodate larger audience members. Boats can no longer take as many passengers as they used to, since the Coast Guard upped its average per-person weight to 185 pounds. And in 2012, one retail chain sold 70,000 bras that were size G (or larger!). Meanwhile, obesity is hitting us at an increasingly younger age: Up to one-third of infants in the United States are now obese or at risk of obesity, according to a study out of Wayne State University.

In fact, the average American circa 2016 who eats the same number of calories and burns off the same number of calories every day still weighs 10 percent more than he or she would have twenty years ago, according to researchers at York University in Canada. And it's not because we're all getting lazy; as a nation, we're exercising more than ever before. But we're still getting fatter.

The main reason can be captured in one word: carbs. We're eating more *carbs* than ever before. Whether they come in the form of fries, pasta, chips, rice, cupcakes, cookies, rolls, muffins, candy, or hundreds of other sources, we're messing up our bodies' natural hormonal systems and creating an almost automatic fat-storage default system.

Those carbs are piling up for three major reasons:

▸ They're everywhere! It used to be that if you wanted to buy a package of Twizzlers, you'd have to go to the local supermarket—or at least a 7-Eleven. But nowadays, Twizzlers are everywhere, including at the checkout at Staples, in giant containers at Costco, and on the checkout line to pay for a hammer at Lowe's. No matter what a store sells nowadays, it also sells carbs. So we're used to grabbing something cheap (and, yes, sometimes tasty) to add on top of whatever else we're shopping for.

▸ They're in *huge* containers! Twenty years ago, a typical portion of soda was 6.5 ounces, according to the National Heart, Lung, and Blood Institute. Today it's 20 ounces— that's the equivalent of 16 teaspoons of sugar. (Check the label on that 20-ounce bottle and chances are it will say "2.5 servings." But I bet you don't really have intentions of splitting it with one and a half other people.) In fact, by 2010 sugary drinks had become the number one source of calories in the American diet, according to the USDA. A quarter of us gets more than 200 calories a day from beverages, and 1 in every 20 Americans gets more than 560 calories! Simply cutting those calories out would save you between 21 and 58 pounds of fat a year.

► The foods are spiked with sugar! Nearly three-quarters of all packaged foods and beverages in the United States have added sugar, according to a 2015 study in *The Lancet Diabetes & Endocrinology*. Next time you're in your kitchen, check out the label of your favorite peanut butter, spaghetti sauce, ketchup, salad dressing, soup, or "healthy" cereal. Chances are, they all have some form of added sugar, whether it's high-fructose corn syrup, cane sugar, agave nectar, turbinado, maltodextrin, barley malt, molasses, or one of dozens of other names that sugar can be listed under. Whether it sounds natural ("wildflower honey") or chemical ("crystalline fructose"), it all has the same effect on our bodies.

When we add sugar to food, we up the carb content, which adds to the impact food has on our weight. And when a packaged food *isn't* high in sugar, it's a good bet that it's high in salt. In both scenarios, an already challenging weight-gain problem is made that much more deadly. A high-carb, low-nutrient diet combines with a lot of sitting and a stressful, often sleep-deprived lifestyle to create a perfect recipe for an obesity epidemic.

Now, it's important that I make clear: 4-Minute Fit is not a plan to fix all of your nutritional problems. Its purpose is to address metabolism. It is what I call nutritional triage. Triage is a term that means "the assignment of degrees of urgency to wounds or illnesses to decide the order of treatment of a large number of patients or casualties." In terms of a battlefield, there are three types of wounded soldiers. There are those whose wounds are so minor that they will be okay even if they don't receive timely medical attention. On the opposite end of the spectrum, there are those soldiers whose wounds are so severe that even if they get medical attention, they are not going to survive. Then there are those in the middle where saving a limb or a life depends on critical, emergency medical care. Those are the soldiers you have to focus on, especially when there are limited resources.

When it comes to your medical condition and nutrition, there may be a whole host of things going on. For my clients, and many readers of this book, the most critical problem is metabolism. By focusing our attention on fixing metabolism, we reduce the risk for the sixty medical disorders and twelve cancers known as metabolic syndrome. So, 4-Minute Fit is a nutritional triage solution for obesity. It has a specific purpose. That is why it is not particularly concerned with sodium intake or cholesterol. Get your metabolism under control first, and then work on other things.

A great way to illustrate this is to consider the case of oatmeal. Lots of people who want to lose weight make the mistake of switching their eggs and bacon breakfast for oatmeal. This is because they heard or think that oatmeal is healthy. Why? Because the American Heart Association says that oatmeal is "heart healthy." It is good for the heart because it lowers cholesterol. So people think, "Oh, oatmeal is healthy. I want to lose weight, so I better eat healthy." And so they start eating oatmeal. But just because something is good for the heart doesn't necessarily mean it's also good for metabolism or losing weight. Just one pack of instant oatmeal has 27 grams of carbohydrates and only 2 grams of protein. So while the oatmeal may lower cholesterol, it is terrible for your metabolism. See the problem here? Some things that are good for your metabolism might not be so good in other areas. Remember, this is nutritional triage!

DIAGNOSING THE DILEMMA

What's causing the obesity problem in the trucking industry is the same thing that's harming all of us. But the way in which the trucking business works makes it a microcosm of our overall society. The weight gain among truckers just happens at a slightly more accelerated pace. As I outline the problem in trucking, take a moment to consider how many similarities exist between this world and your own busy, sedentary, stress-filled life.

It starts with the drivers' irregular schedules and interrupted sleep, which accumulates every day and creates chronic sleep deprivation. This, in turn, affects serum leptin and ghrelin production, which hinders proper metabolism and hunger regulation. This causes drivers to either skip meals (slowing the body's metabolism) or overeat, especially carb-heavy junk food (leading to fat storage).

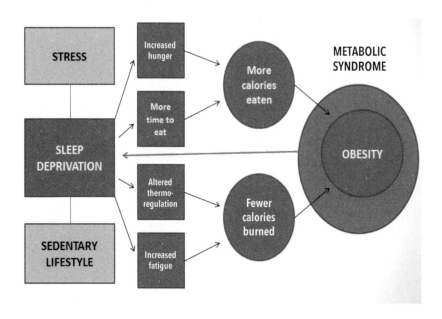

THE VICIOUS CYCLE

In either case, the average driver is getting only about *one-third* of the nutrition he needs every day in the form of protein, fiber, vitamins, and minerals. Meanwhile, whether he is overeating (because there is so much food available) or undereating (because he's too busy or stressed, or he's "trying to lose weight"), the poor quality of his diet causes him to become deficient in many different nutrients, especially B vitamins (found in beans, leafy greens, poultry, and fish) as well as the critical minerals calcium and magnesium (which come from many of the same sources, as well as from dairy products). This in turn decreases the body's ability to handle what is already a very stressful job. The resulting vitamin and mineral deficiencies trigger sweet and salty food cravings and a "stress eating" reflex. Meanwhile, the stress hormone cortisol is chronically flooding and coursing through the driver's system, causing fat storage and drawing blood flow away from the major internal organs, depriving them of the nutrition they need. Ultimately, the body becomes increasingly stressed, the hormones become increasingly imbalanced, and fat storage and insulin insensitivity—the beginning stage of diabetes—increase. In addition, studies have shown that when people miss out on vitamins, minerals, and other crucial nutrients, the damage goes right down to their DNA. In fact, drivers trapped in a junk-food cycle may suffer damage to their DNA that mimics damage caused by radiation. (This DNA damage is called *epigenetics*, which refers to permanent changes in our genetic makeup caused by environmental factors. A 2014 study at Leiden University in the Netherlands found that poor nutrition not only can damage our own bodies but can change our DNA in a way that causes us to pass this damage down to future generations!)

This cycle is so common that I went so far as to outline "Nine Steps of Creating an Unhealthy, Unsafe Driver":

1. In the first week of a driver's career, the stress of learning how to drive a truck and of starting a new job will often increase cortisol levels, initiating the first hormonal change.

2. In the next two to four weeks, the irregular schedule (and frequently interrupted sleep) results in accumulated sleep deprivation. This does much more than make us feel groggy and lacking in sharpness. After just four nights of sleep deprivation, insulin sensitivity drops by as much as 16 percent and fat cell sensitivity to insulin drops by 30 percent. This is the equivalent of metabolically aging someone *ten to twenty years* just from four nights of partial sleep restriction.

3. After four weeks of passively sitting in the driver's seat during a regular driving shift, the hip flexors—muscles that connect the hips to the knee—tighten and shorten, causing bad posture and improper force loading on the joints, leading to ankle, knee, hip, lower back, neck, and shoulder injuries. (Adding insult to injury, tight hip flexors also cause the pelvis to tip forward in a way that makes your belly look bigger than it actually is.)

4. After three months, the driver's serum leptin and serum ghrelin levels have been altered, and the driver's body is unable to regulate hunger properly. Glucose reserves in the liver and muscle are full and the body can no longer store excess carbohydrates as anything but fat.

5. By this time, the vast majority of drivers will start skipping meals in order to keep the truck rolling. As the body goes into starvation mode, low leptin levels signal to the brain that the body needs feeding. Energy expenditure is reduced to compensate for the lack of food intake, thus *lowering metabolism*. This creates a hormonal environment conducive to storing fat. Thyroid hormones fall, while cortisol and ghrelin hormones rise. The combined effect of these hormonal changes is a lower metabolism and an increase in appetite and fat storage. So the driver both starves himself *and* overeats when he finally does get a meal. Talk about a worst-case scenario! (And—literally—a potentially deadly combination.)

6. After six months on the job, the average driver has gained significant body fat and lost lean muscle. This combination decreases the body's ability to extract oxygen from the blood at the cellular level. That's a problem, because the body uses oxygen to produce a compound called *adenosine triphosphate* (ATP). ATP is to the body what money is to the economy: It pretty much fuels and kick-starts everything that's happening inside of you, so the less you have, the less you can accomplish. With decreased levels of ATP, there is less usable energy on hand. The result is that the driver feels more fatigued and has less energy available for the activities of daily living and truck driving.

7. From six months to one year on the job, a truck driver has now gained a full 7 percent of his body weight on average and added 1 inch to his waist. He has increased his risk for

sixty medical disorders including twelve cancers. Specifically,

- ► Blood pressure increases by 10 percent

- ► Blood cholesterol level increases by 8 percent

- ► High-density lipoprotein (HDL) decreases by 15 percent

- ► Triglycerides increase by 18 percent

- ► Metabolic syndrome risk increases by 18 percent

8. Once the driver becomes "obese"—that is, his fat increases and his muscle decreases until he reaches a BMI of more than 30.0—things get even worse. The average truck driver in America (about 69 percent of us on the road) has a threefold increase in the above numbers.

9. Once the driver is obese, he has a 20 to 30 percent greater likelihood of developing severe obstructive sleep apnea. And once that happens, the driver has a sevenfold increased risk of being involved in a motor vehicle accident. Obese drivers with sleep apnea cause 45 percent more accidents per mile driven than nonobese drivers with no sleep-disordered breathing. This is another example of the obesity causing collateral damage and horrible indirect results to go with its horrible direct results.

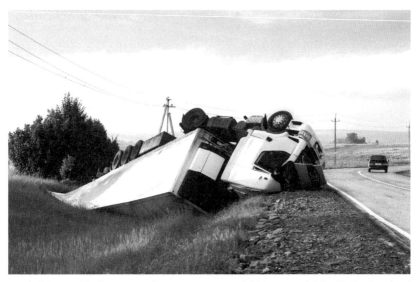

Truck drivers with sleep apnea have up to a sevenfold increased risk of being involved in a motor vehicle crash. (*Science Daily*, March 12, 2009)

THE BELLY FAT CYCLE

As you can see, eating too little has the same end effect as eating too much: a disrupted hormonal system, a lowered metabolism, and fat storage.

That fat storage happens primarily in the form of visceral fat cells, or belly fat. When your body needs to store fat, it doesn't necessarily create new fat cells; instead, it makes the fat cells you do have grow larger to accommodate the increase in lipids that each cell has to store.

As the individual fat cells swell, they become more active, sending out greater and greater levels of adipokines. As you saw in a previous chapter, these raised levels cause more inflammation, which further damages your hormonal system, making you crave more carbs, which you then eat, creating more fat storage and giving your belly fat even more power. Your belly fat basically "tricks" you into helping it grow.

What we need, then, is a plan to keep us exercising and eating regularly—so we're not underfed, slowing our metabolism, or constantly hungry, causing us to overeat. But we also need to be eating the right stuff—so we keep feeding our bodies the nutrients it needs and we always feel full and satisfied.

Fortunately, the solution is pretty simple. In the next chapters, I'll outline how a smart exercising and eating schedule will shrink your belly rapidly and return your hormones and metabolism back to their proper levels.

How Your Belly Bugs Make You Fat

On any given day, there may be as many as 3.5 million truckers on the roads, highways, and byways of the United States. Some truckers are hauling diesel, some are trucking produce, some might have loads of lawn chairs or cake mix or cement. But each of them has a job to do, and the economy simply does not run unless those jobs get done.

In many ways, your GI tract is a lot like America's highways. Except there is even more going on: trillions of microbes patrol your digestive system, with more than five hundred different species doing things like helping to break down food, kill off invading bacteria, and managing your hormonal system.

Our belly biome evolved to eat a particular type of diet, and one of the reasons we have such an exploding obesity problem is that the food we're feeding our microscopic army isn't supporting them in the way they need. Our diets are much too high in simple carbohydrates like white rice, bread, pasta, and sugar, and too low in protein, healthy fats, and fiber. Since different bugs do different jobs, that just throws the balance of our biome out of whack.

To take the trucking metaphor to its extreme, imagine we sent out five times as many trucks hauling paint, but never sent any trucks carrying brushes. You'd have a whole lot of stores wondering what to do with all those cans of paint, and a whole lot of customers who couldn't get their chores done because there were no brushes to use. The whole construction industry would slow to a standstill.

The same thing happens when you feed your belly too much junk food and not enough protein, fiber, vitamins, and minerals. Bacteria that feed off sugar and carbs get much stronger, overwhelming the other gut bugs that are supposed to balance them out. This leads to inflammation and what's known as a "leaky gut"—basically, the fine mesh screen that lines your digestive system becomes porous and inflamed, and bacteria and other toxins leak into your body, causing more inflammation and greater fat storage. (In studies, obese people have higher levels of a bacteria type known as Firmicutes, while those who are thinner tend to have higher levels of a good bacteria called Bacteroidetes.) It's not unlike what happens to your gums if you eat a lot of starchy, sugary foods and don't brush your teeth: the bacteria in your mouth thrive on the sugar, and your gums get red and inflamed. Too much of that and your teeth start falling out. Diabetes and heart disease are both closely linked to the sort of inflammation that can stem from a leaky gut.

But when your gut health is disrupted, it also means you're not getting as much nutrition out of the meals you do eat. That's because the microbes in your gut help to digest your food and pull nutrients out of it. When your digestive biome balance is off, you get even less nutrition from the foods you do eat, and that means that less of what you eat winds up being used for fuel—another factor in weight gain.

Four Reasons to Swear Off Soda

I believe in freedom, all kinds of freedom. But I want to discuss now a specific kind of freedom that I hold dear: food freedom. That is, the ability to eat what you want and make your own choices. I make it a policy not to ban any food or drink from my clients' diets. My goal is to get you to make small, gradual changes that, over time, have enormous effect. But if there's one change you can make today that will have a dramatic impact on your health and your appearance, it's giving up soda, sweet tea, energy drinks, sports drinks, juice, and other beverages that come with sugar or high fructose corn syrup in them. The next time you're deciding what to wash down your meal with, here are four reasons why unsweetened soft drinks, sparkling water, or good old tap water are a better choice than a soda or an iced tea:

- ► You'll drop pounds. One study followed 200,000 people over twenty years and found that those who drank just one more sugary drink per day weighed at average of five pounds more than those who did not.
- ► You'll protect your family. Here's a reason not to make soda drinking a habit: for each 12-ounce sweetened beverage a child consumes per day, his or her risk of becoming obese over the next eighteen months increases by 60 percent, according to a study in *The Lancet*.
- ► You'll reduce your diabetes risk. People who consume just one or two sugary drinks a day have a 26 percent greater risk of diabetes than those who don't, according to a *Diabetes Care* study.
- ► You'll help strengthen your heart. A study that followed 40,000 men for twenty years found that those who drank

just one can of a sugary beverage a day had a 20 percent higher risk of dying from heart attack than those who drank none. (I should add that this includes diet soda, which, studies reveal, more people drink at work than regular soda. Yes, you're saving yourself the 140 calories. But the artificial sweetener triggers insulin, which can set your body into fat storage mode and lead to weight gain.)

6 How to Make 4-Minute Fit Work for You

Now that you're on your way to tracking your exercise and getting comfortable with a daily routine, we can add the food component. One of the major problems with most diets is that, by nature, they're temporary. You "go on a diet," and then, of course, you "go off" the diet. That's why this plan doesn't have lists of "forbidden foods" or "super foods" that you need to eat every day, or points or rules or other complicated structures. Instead of changing the food you eat, my goal is to change the way you think about eating.

This is called *nutritional cognitive restructuring*. Those are big, expensive words for a pretty simple concept: once you become more aware of the way you eat, it becomes much easier to make smart choices that will boost your metabolism and rev up your natural fat burners.

I can't overstate the impact of simply being thoughtful about what you eat. In 2016, researchers at the University of California San Francisco put 200 obese people on identical eating and exercise programs. But half of the group got general stress relief counseling, while the other half was taught about mindful eating—essentially, being present and aware of the food they were consuming, rather than just blindly following the diet protocol. While both groups lost similar amounts of weight during the trial, researchers found that six months later, the mindful-eating group had much better long-term results, including healthier cholesterol profiles and lower blood sugar levels. Their metabolisms were faster and healthier.

Changing the way you eat is hard if you don't change the way you think first. That's what this plan will do for you.

Are you ready to get going? Here's where the instructions begin!

HOW TO TRACK, AND MASTER, YOUR NUTRITION

Most of us make food choices based on circumstances, convenience, economics, habit, and hearsay. We don't generally make food choices based on the nutritional content of the food we eat or the effect that food will have on metabolism. Logging and tracking food changes that. The more you track nutrition, the more you start to learn the nutritional content of the food you eat. You want to shift from thinking, "What sounds good to eat today?" to "What can I eat now that is going to have a positive effect on my metabolism?" Fortunately, the vast majority of us now have access to a smartphone, which can make tracking nutrition throughout the day remarkably easy and provide us with instant feedback on our choices. When you track your nutrition as you eat throughout the day, you can also keep a running tab on your carb intake to help determine what you can and cannot afford to eat later in the day. This is the first step in taking control of your food, and so for the first week, this is what we'll concentrate on.

WEEK ONE

Download Your App

Not all that long ago, in order to track nutrition, you had to have a pen or pencil, a piece of paper, and some reference material. You would write down what you ate and then spend time figuring out the serving size and looking through reference materials to find the amount of calories, fats, carbs, protein, and so on, you had just consumed. If you wanted to know your totals for the day, or anything else, you had to do a lot of math.

Today? Logging nutrition couldn't be easier. There are hundreds of online tools and smartphone apps that make logging, measuring, and tracking food easy and quick. While any food logging program or app will suffice, I recommend for my clients MyFitnessPal for ease of use. There's a free version, it has a great food database, and logging food is relatively easy. (MyFitnessPal can also read bar codes from food packages, a feature people really like.)

For more serious clients, I also recommend Cronometer, for its micronutrient tracking capability and overall nutritional analysis. It costs $2.99 but also allows for micronutrient tracking, which few apps do. No matter which product you use, the fundamentals are all the same. Other apps that people have used with success include MyFoodDiary, LoseIt!, FatSecret, and SparkPeople. Bottom line: we are all lucky to live at a time when technology makes our lives easier in so many ways. Devices and apps that enable us to track our nutrition—and then enable us to see our weaknesses and strengths so we can formulate a plan—are an absolute gift. In our war against obesity, this is high-tech weaponry. We should take advantage of it!

Begin Your Food Log

The goal of the first week is simply to establish your profile and get comfortable with the app and the technology. There is a learning curve when tracking your nutrition, and for some, this can be more challenging than for others. That's normal.

Once you're comfortable, log everything you eat and drink for the next seven days. It is very important that you *do not change any eating habits*! Eat normally—do not try to make changes or impress the new fitness trainer. Once you complete the seven-day food log, the first thing you will want to do is determine your average daily meal frequency. How often did you eat? Your goal after the first week is to increase your meal frequency. For maximum results, you want to eat five times a day, spaced at three-hour intervals.

Generally speaking, I divide the day into breakfast, morning snack, lunch, afternoon snack, dinner, and late snack. (*Snack* is a term that resists definition as far as I'm concerned, but it's purposefully lighter than a meal. Also, we're trained to think of "snack" as a negative term, but I'd encourage you to think of it as an important part of daily nourishing.) For each day, add up the number of meals and snacks consumed or the number of times you ate. Then add the total for each of the seven days and divide by 7. This will give you average daily meal frequency. Whatever the number is, you want to set a Week 2 goal that is a little better.

Remember, in Week 1 all we're doing is establishing your baseline. We are figuring out where you are now and where you want to go. That is the key. Don't make any changes to your nutrition. Just learn how to log your food and establish your nutrition profile. A nutritional log answers questions like:

- ▶ What is my average daily calorie intake?

- ▶ What is my daily average carbohydrate intake?

> ► What's my daily average protein intake?

> ► What's my meal frequency?

You can use any food logging program that you want as long as it shows you your calories, your carbohydrates, and your proteins, and lets you calculate your meal frequency—meaning when you eat your food, it goes under breakfast, snack, lunch, snack, dinner. If you are not part of twenty-first-century technology, that's cool. Just write down the information by hand,

A typical food log looks like this:

Breakfast		
Ionix Supreme	1 Serving	25
IsaLean Pro French Vanilla Shake	1 × 1 Packet	280
Blueberries, wild, frozen	1 cup, whole pieces	71.4
Ageless Essentials with 4th Generation Product B AM Pack	1 g	0
bicycling, to/from work, self selected pace	15 minutes	-101.93
Omelet, made with onion, tomato, peppers, mushrooms	3 medium egg used - 1 whole egg or 2 egg whites	373.21
AM Snack		
Almonds, raw	10 each	71.39
Lunch		
Clif Builder's 20g Protein Bar, Chocolate Peanut Butter	1 bar - each 2.4 oz	263.47
Starbucks Refreshers Raspberry Pomegranate	1 oz	7.5
PM Snack		
Simple Squares Coconut Honey Bar	0.5 Serving	115
Original Living Coconut Vanilla Bean Coconut Cream Dessert	0.2 × 1 serving	29
Ageless Essentials with 4th Generation Product B PM Pack	1 g	0
Chocolate chip cookies, bakery	0.5 each - approx 2 1/4" diameter	38.96
Dinner		
Gyro sandwich	0.44 sandwich	356.74

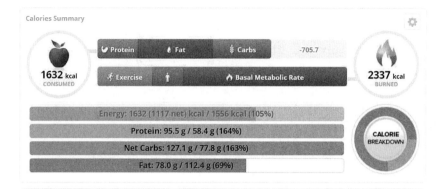

Calories Summary

1632 kcal CONSUMED

Protein · Fat · Carbs · -705.7

Exercise · Basal Metabolic Rate

2337 kcal BURNED

Energy: 1632 (1117 net) kcal / 1556 kcal (105%)
Protein: 95.5 g / 58.4 g (164%)
Net Carbs: 127.1 g / 77.8 g (163%)
Fat: 78.0 g / 112.4 g (69%)

CALORIE BREAKDOWN

Nutrient Targets

| 95% TARGETS | 82% Carbs | 303% Zinc | 370% Selenium | 129% Magnesium | 1183% Vit.D | 81% Calcium | 133% Omega-3 |

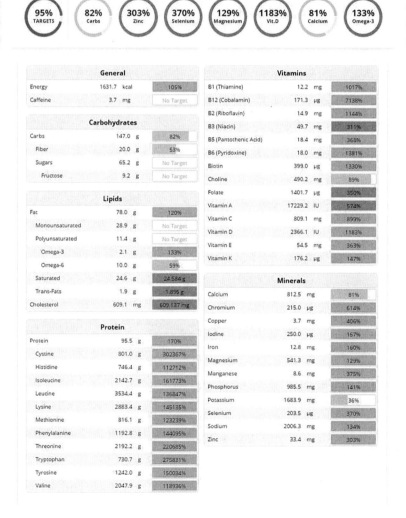

General			
Energy	1631.7	kcal	105%
Caffeine	3.7	mg	No Target

Carbohydrates			
Carbs	147.0	g	82%
Fiber	20.0	g	53%
Sugars	65.2	g	No Target
Fructose	9.2	g	No Target

Lipids			
Fat	78.0	g	120%
Monounsaturated	28.9	g	No Target
Polyunsaturated	11.4	g	No Target
Omega-3	2.1	g	133%
Omega-6	10.0	g	59%
Saturated	24.6	g	24.584 g
Trans-Fats	1.9	g	1.895 g
Cholesterol	609.1	mg	609.137 mg

Protein			
Protein	95.5	g	170%
Cystine	801.0	g	302367%
Histidine	746.4	g	112712%
Isoleucine	2142.7	g	161773%
Leucine	3534.4	g	136847%
Lysine	2883.4	g	145135%
Methionine	816.1	g	123239%
Phenylalanine	1192.8	g	144095%
Threonine	2192.2	g	220685%
Tryptophan	730.7	g	275831%
Tyrosine	1242.0	g	150034%
Valine	2047.9	g	118936%

Vitamins			
B1 (Thiamine)	12.2	mg	1017%
B12 (Cobalamin)	171.3	µg	7138%
B2 (Riboflavin)	14.9	mg	1144%
B3 (Niacin)	49.7	mg	311%
B5 (Pantothenic Acid)	18.4	mg	368%
B6 (Pyridoxine)	18.0	mg	1381%
Biotin	399.0	µg	1330%
Choline	490.2	mg	89%
Folate	1401.7	µg	350%
Vitamin A	17229.2	IU	574%
Vitamin C	809.1	mg	899%
Vitamin D	2366.1	IU	1183%
Vitamin E	54.5	mg	363%
Vitamin K	176.2	µg	147%

Minerals			
Calcium	812.5	mg	81%
Chromium	215.0	µg	614%
Copper	3.7	mg	406%
Iodine	250.0	µg	167%
Iron	12.8	mg	160%
Magnesium	541.3	mg	129%
Manganese	8.6	mg	375%
Phosphorus	985.5	mg	141%
Potassium	1683.9	mg	36%
Selenium	203.5	µg	370%
Sodium	2006.3	mg	134%
Zinc	33.4	mg	303%

WEEK TWO

Hit Your Five-a-Day Goal

In Week 2, we're going to concentrate on meal frequency. The sooner you get to 5.0 meals a day (35 meals a week), the sooner you'll maximize your results. Five meals entail breakfast, a late-morning snack, lunch, an afternoon snack, and dinner. That's the minimum level to get maximum results, because you *must* feed, or "fuel," your metabolism every three hours so it doesn't turn off. (Once you start a fire, you've got to keep putting logs on it to keep it going, right? You've got to make sure every three hours you put a new log on the fire of your metabolism to keep it going, or you're just going to let it burn out.)

Cut Your Carbs

This week we're also going to start cutting carbohydrates. Remember, a main nutritional goal of 4-Minute Fit is the gradual reduction of carbohydrates in order to limit the amount of glucose available for producing energy and being stored as fat while instead promoting the burning of fat. Perhaps the most important nutrition metric, then, is the average daily carbohydrate consumption.

For each day, record the total number of carbohydrates consumed. Then add the daily total for each of the seven days to get the total number of carbohydrates consumed for the week and divide that number by 7 to get the average daily carbohydrate consumption. Whatever that number is, you want to reduce that number gradually each week. As a rule, you'll aim for a reduction of somewhere between 5 percent and 10 percent. If your average daily carbohydrate consumption was between 300 and 350 grams, your goal for Week 2 is to cut 20 to 25 grams of carbs from your average daily intake. How you do that? Simple. Look at your food log from Week 1 and highlight any-thing you eat that has more than 20 grams of carbs. Some examples:

- ▶ French fries

- ▶ Potato chips

- ▶ Most granola bars

- ▶ Bananas

- ▶ Pizza

- ▶ Sodas and many juices

Which of those items did you consume the most? Let's target those. One trick: substitute your beverages. It's likely going to be easier to replace your root beer or iced tea with water than it is to replace your chips with a different food. (It's entirely possible that you're drink-ing, not eating, one-fourth—even one-third—of your carbs every day.)

Here are the ranges I recommend:

CARBOHYDRATE LEVEL	REDUCE BY
more than 300g carbs	20 to 25g for the next week
200 to 300g carbs	15 to 20g for the next week
140 to 200g carbs	10 to 15g for the next week

For example, if your Week 1 average daily carbohydrate consump-tion was 320 grams, you will set a goal for Week 2 at 295 to 300 grams.

Each week you'll reset the goal by reducing another 15 grams to 20 grams. So if you get to 295 grams during Week 2, then for Week 3, you'll set a goal of 275 to 280 grams. You'll keep reducing by 15 to 20 grams until you reach an average daily carbohydrate consumption of 200 grams.

From there, you'll set a new goal of reducing consumption by 10 to 15 grams a week until you get to 140 grams. At that point, you do not need to continue reducing carbs, and it becomes all about maintenance.

Once you have this information in hand, you can analyze: what is the thing you eat most frequently that does the most damage to your metabolism? Look at any food that has 20 grams of carbs or more and highlight it. I had one driver who loved Subway's foot-long subs and would eat four or five of them a week. Well, each of those subs have more than 80 grams of carbs. I had another driver who drank eighteen Mountain Dews a week. Well, each 20-ounce bottle of Mountain Dew packs 77 grams of carbs.

A third driver told me he liked granola bars. "It's only one hundred calories, better than chips and Doritos," he reckoned, not unreasonably. He ate four granola bars a day, twenty-eight each week. The problem is that granola bars are so heavy on carbs. I didn't tell him to stop eating granola bars. I told him to switch from Kellogg's Special K granola bars to Nature Valley Protein Chewy bars. "It's basically the same product and flavor, but the one I am encouraging you to eat has ten fewer grams of carbs. If you eat four a day, you're cutting forty grams. That's basically ten percent of your intake right there."

Swap In Protein

Carbs undermine your metabolic function, because they're digested quickly and they're packed with energy—energy your body is forced to store as fat. Protein, on the other hand, is a key driver of metabolism. Protein helps fire up your fat burners in two ways. First, it's the building block of muscle, and the more muscle you have, the greater your metabolism. Muscle burns energy on a regular basis, so it steals energy away from fat cells—specifically belly fat cells—in order to sustain itself. Your belly fat just hates the idea of your muscles storing energy (in the form of glycogen) that could otherwise be used to make more fat cells. (You'll read more about why building muscle is so important a little later in this chapter.)

Second, the very act of eating protein actually burns calories. About 25 percent of the calories you eat in the form of protein are burned up just digesting the protein itself (carbs and fat burn up no more than 10 to 15 percent of their calories). A 2012 study in the *International Journal of Obesity* found that obese adults who ate three servings of protein-packed yogurt each day as part of a reduced-calorie diet lost 22 percent more weight and 61 percent more body fat compared to those who didn't have the yogurt.

Protein also keeps you fuller longer—in part because that intense digestive process means your body perceives you as being satiated. In a 2013 study in the journal *Appetite*, women were fed low-, medium-, or high-protein afternoon snacks. Those who ate the most protein had the lowest levels of hunger and waited longer before they chose to eat again than those who ate lower-protein snacks. In part, that's because of our hormonal response to protein. Another study published in the *American Journal of Clinical Nutrition* found that a high-protein meal, as opposed to one high in carbs, increases satiety by suppressing the hunger-stimulating hormone ghrelin.

And switching to a higher-protein diet helps you build a base that will keep you burning calories for life. In a study in the *International Journal of Obesity*, researchers found that dieters who ate a low-calorie, high-protein diet for eight weeks lost an average of 24 pounds. But unlike those in the trial who ate a low-protein, low-calorie diet, those in the high-protein group continued to lose weight, an average of 5 percent more, after the study was over. And after six months, the high-protein group had kept all of their weight off.

WEEK THREE

Determine Your Average Daily Calorie Consumption

Just as you did with carbohydrates, determine your average daily calorie consumption. For each day, record the total number of calories you consumed. Then add the daily total for each of the seven days to get the total number of calories consumed for the week and divide that number by 7 to get the average daily calorie consumption.

This step isn't about reducing the amount of food you eat. It's about making sure you're eating enough while still reducing your carb intake. Sometimes when we cut out the big-carb items, we don't always do a good job of replacing them with high-protein alternatives, and our calorie intake drops. That's unhealthy. When it comes to losing weight, I have found that men get the best results between 1,700 and 2,000 calories while women get the best results between 1,500 and 1,700 calories. However, because the vast majority of people have been programmed to think that the best way to lose weight is to restrict calories, they try to count calories and keep them as low as possible. This is especially true for women. Don't do that!

Remember, 4-Minute Fit is not about calorie counting. More important than reducing calories—which has very little to do with metabolism and hormones—is monitoring and reducing carbohydrates. If you are not getting enough nutrition, the body will go into starvation mode and try to hold on to fat instead of burn it. Count carbs, *not* calories!

Why There's No Such Thing as "Cheating"

Most weight-loss plans require you to swear off certain foods entirely, except for certain "cheat meals" or "cheat days." Living a life of deprivation sucks. And it's not conducive to motivating someone or to sustaining long-term success. That's why 4-Minute Fit is designed to allow for food freedom. When you are free to eat whatever you want, you feel good. Once you establish your nutritional profile or baseline, you can then look at your average daily carbohydrate consumption. If it's high, then the goal for the next week is to reduce it enough to have a metabolic effect, but not so much that it provokes an adverse effect like food cravings.

So let's say the goal is to reduce your average daily carbohydrate consumption by 10 grams. Does that mean you can't ever eat French fries or a chocolate chip cookie? That you can never eat a cheeseburger? Of course not. What you will learn is when and how to eat those foods you love. For example, if you eat an unhealthy, carb-loaded breakfast like oatmeal with a banana and a glass of orange juice—a breakfast with anywhere between 70 grams and 100 grams of carbs—then you have spent your carb budget early in the day. (Yes, I just said that a breakfast of oatmeal, banana, and orange juice is *unhealthy* if weight loss is your goal! More on that later.) That means that on that day, you can't afford to eat your spaghetti with garlic bread for dinner. Doing so will put you over your carb budget. So instead you choose the grilled chicken salad in order to bring your carb intake under control.

Now, if you're going to Olive Garden for dinner and you want that spaghetti and garlic bread, then you plan for it by managing the first half of your day. You have a carb-light breakfast (less than 30 grams—think a nice plate of scrambled eggs), a carb-light snack (less than 10 grams), a carb-light lunch (less than 30 grams—maybe a soup and a salad), and a carb-light snack (less than 10 grams). That's only 80 grams of carbs. Now you have enough in your carb budget to afford the spaghetti and garlic bread. Or maybe you have enough for the spaghetti only, so you skip the garlic bread.

In this way, you're free to eat anything you like and still get weight-loss results. This is the benefit of having a "system" based on balancing nutritional content, not on trying to avoid certain "bad" foods.

Using the Nutrition Log

Keeping a nutrition log is essential to this program, because it gives you an objective reference from which you can begin to change your diet. Each week, here is what you want to do:

1. Identify items with 40 grams of carbs or more. Two slices of bread have about 44 grams of carbs. So does a large baked potato. A package of Little Debbies will get you near 40 as well. If you eat an item with 40 grams of carbs once or twice a week, consider it an indulgence. But anything you eat more frequently than that should be cut out.

2. Identify *frequently eaten* items with 20 grams or more of carbs and less than 8 grams of protein, and calculate the total sum of each. A slice of fast-food thin-crust pizza, for example, has 24 grams of carbs and just 9 grams of protein.

3. Calculate the percentage of average daily carb consumption of the top three items from Step 2.

4. Identify substitutions for items from Step 3 and calculate the reduction in carbs to show why this is going to work. Generally, it's these everyday foods, not the occasional indulgences, that do us in.

5. Gradually reduce carbs systematically in this fashion until you reach 125 grams to 140 grams carbs per day (In many cases, a 25 percent reduction in carbs is sufficient for average results.)

Let's look at an example using MyFitnessPal. Below is a nutrition log for two of the seven days.

May 13, 2015

FOODS	Calories	Carbs	Fat	Protein	Cholest	Sodium	Sugars	Fiber
Breakfast								
Kellogg's® - Pop-tarts - Frosted Strawberry, 2 Pastry (52g)	400	76g	10g	4g	0mg	340mg	32g	2g
Lunch								
Nissin Chow Mein - Chicken Flavor, 1 container	480	70g	18g	12g	0mg	1,340mg	16g	4g
Dinner								
Walmart - Walmart Meat Lovers Pizza, 2 slice	720	54g	38g	34g	100mg	1,820mg	6g	2g
Snacks								
Mountain Dew - Baja Blast, 20 oz	280	73g	0g	0g	0mg	75mg	73g	0g
Yvonne's Casa - Sweet Seedless Red Grapes, 1 cup	104	27g	0g	0g	0mg	3mg	23g	1g
Kellogg's® - Pop-tarts - Frosted Strawberry, 2 Pastry (52g)	400	76g	10g	4g	0mg	340mg	32g	2g
Planter's - Dry Roasted Peanuts, 6 oz (about 39 pieces)	960	30g	84g	42g	0mg	900mg	12g	12g
TOTAL:	3,344	406g	160g	96g	100mg	4,818mg	194g	23g

EXERCISES			Calories	Minutes	Sets	Reps	Weight
Cardiovascular							
Garmin Connect calorie adjustment			44	1			
TOTALS:			44	1	0	0	0

May 14, 2015

FOODS	Calories	Carbs	Fat	Protein	Cholest	Sodium	Sugars	Fiber
Breakfast								
Kellogg's - Pop-Tarts - Frosted Strawberry, 2 Pastry	400	76g	10g	4g	0mg	340mg	32g	2g
Dinner								
Stouffer's - Deluxe French Bread Pizza, 2 Pizza	840	88g	42g	28g	60mg	1,640mg	12g	4g
Snacks								
Herr's - Peanut Butter Pretzels, 9 pieces	140	15g	7g	5g	0mg	330mg	2g	2g
Herr's - Peanut Butter Pretzels, 9 pieces	140	15g	7g	5g	0mg	330mg	2g	2g
Campbell's Chunky - Sirloin Burger With Country Vegetables, 1 container (2 cups ea.)	280	34g	10g	14g	40mg	1,580mg	6g	6g
Hickory Harvest - Island Fruit Mix, 1/4 cup	105	26g	0g	0g	0mg	48mg	22g	1g
Stouffers - Baked Ziti, 1 pkg (453g)	520	68g	18g	22g	50mg	1,100mg	13g	5g
TOTAL:	2,425	322g	94g	78g	150mg	5,368mg	89g	22g

This is the nutrition log review I sent to this client:

Greetings,

Okay, below is your food log, and I have circled in red the items that are really causing damage. Remember, you don't have to change everything all at once. I am going to show you step by step what to change. Also remember this: when you eat foods with a lot of carbohydrates (more than 20 grams) and your body doesn't need the energy at that time (because you are sitting down driving and not doing much), your body converts the carbs into fat and stores it in your body. So look at the foods you have been eating below that are circled in red and look at the amount of carbs. From your food log, your average daily carb consumption is 325.5 grams. That's high. What's the single biggest offender? You had Pop-Tarts eight times for a total of 663 grams, or an average of 83 grams per day. That's 25.5 percent of your daily carb consumption. At 5'10" and 263 pounds, and with a BMI of 38 and employed in the unhealthiest occupation in America, you cannot afford to be eating like this. So here is what you do. Stop at Walmart and buy two boxes of Nature Valley Protein Chewy Bars. There are five in a box, so that's ten bars. Each bar has just 14 grams of carbs and 10 grams of protein, so it is one of the very best snacks for your metabolism. Stop buying the Pop-Tarts and eat two of the protein bars instead (total of 28 grams of carbs). That one change alone will reduce your carbs by 55 grams per day or down to a total of 270.5 grams of carbs per day. That's a 17 percent improvement from just one change alone. Focus on that and let's get your average daily carbs down to 270 grams. That's enough to give your body a metabolic boost. Once you do that, I will show you the next step.

The same way we are working on making these incremental gains in exercises, you should be doing with nutrition. Your baseline was 2.7 meals a day? This week you should try and improve that by 10 percent. Get to 3.0 or, for that psychic payoff, 3.1. If you were skipping breakfast some days and just eating lunch and dinner, it's unrealistic to go from that to suddenly eating five small meals. But just making sure to eat breakfast will get you to a meal frequency of 3.0. Some clients can go straight to 5.0 meals. If so, that's great!

These gains will work synergistically with the exercises. Combining a little improvement in nutrition with a little improvement in exercise will amplify results. Consistency is the key.

So now you have created a new exercise program for yourself, and you've created a nutrition plan for yourself. Both are based on the things you love, and you've customized them to fit your lifestyle. That's part of the magic of 4-Minute Fit: No one's diet and exercise plan will be exactly like yours. Because no one is exactly like you!

4-MINUTE MYTH BUSTER

"Eating late at night will cause weight gain."

WRONG!

A common belief is that when we eat at night, and then go to sleep, our bodies store the food we just ate as fat, because we're not moving around and burning off those recently consumed calories. Completely false. To keep your metabolism running high and your fat-burners working optimally, it's important to eat five meals and spread your food intake throughout the day, focusing on protein and cutting down on carbs. The calories of a food don't change based on what time of day it is or what time of day it's eaten. Neither does the body's determination of which calories will be stored as fat and which will be burned. We all keep different hours. If you have a late shift and don't get to dinner until late at night, that's fine. If you work out late at night, it is essential to eat and drink after your session, replacing the nutrients and water you have just lost in the gym. Fuel your body!

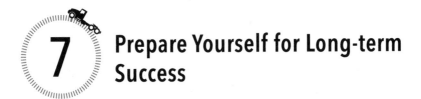

7 Prepare Yourself for Long-term Success

USING THE 4-MINUTE WORKSHEET TO SPARK YOUR MOTIVATION

You've read about the incredible improvements you can make in your life in just four minutes a day.

You've read about the dangerous, damaging consequences of not making those changes.

And you've read how easy it is to get started, with a quick, simple exercise program you can do anywhere and a customized diet that's built around the foods you already love to eat.

But if you're still reading, and not acting, it's probably because intellectually you're ready for a change. But emotionally you're not quite there yet.

That's the purpose of this chapter. To prepare you for getting over that hump, to go from "I should . . ." to "I did!"

JUMP-START YOUR MOTIVATION

If you're like most people starting this program, you're going from nothing to something. You haven't been working out. You haven't been following a nutritional program. And now you're going to start. That's great. Congratulations! There are never any judgments here. Just making the decision that you need to make a change? That's a strong first step.

The beginning stages of this plan—the first four weeks or so—are the buildup phase. You'll be working on your nutritional intake, analyzing it to determine which of the foods you're putting in your body are doing the most damage. There is no diet to "go on," and there are no strict rules regarding foods that you must eat, or must avoid, every day.

Your workout plan, too, is flexible and based around your lifestyle, your fitness level, and the exercises you're comfortable with. What can you change or add to your daily routine—one thing at a time—so you can exercise vigorously? By the end of the first four weeks, your fitness is going to be noticeably improved, plus your better nutrition is going to start having an effect. But before we do anything, some self-analysis is critical. People often say in the beginning, "What should I be eating? Is this food good for me? How many of these should I have? What exercise should I begin with?"

Think of it this way: If you ask me, *How do I get to New York?* I can try and give you an answer. But first, I need to know where you are. If you're in Boston, it's one set of instructions. If you're in Denver, it's another. If it's Florida, it's an entirely different path. How can I give you meaningful instructions or meaningful directions when I don't know your starting point? So this chapter is about helping you understand your starting point, and making you ready to begin the first leg of your fitness journey.

SETTING YOUR PRIORITIES

By the time most drivers get to me, they are desperate. Diagnosed with this or that condition, afraid of losing their Department of Transportation certification—or worse yet, not being around for their families—these drivers are ready to change. They just want to know what to do. When my drivers show up the first day, committed to losing weight and changing their lifestyle, I start by asking them a series of questions.

The first one is simple:

> ▶ What is the most important thing in your life?

Now I'm asking *you*. Write down an answer or at least just consider the question. The answers vary, but you can probably guess the common response. It's "family" or some variation—my kids, my spouse, my partner, my parents. Surely you've heard the saying "People are more important than things." Here's proof. For as long as I've been asking this question, no one has responded "my car" or "my boat" or even "my house."

A follow-up question:

> ▶ Can you take care of the most important feature of your life—your family—if you are sick, in the hospital, or can't hold down a job?

The inevitable answer is no. Good health is the *prerequisite* for having and keeping a job and taking care of one's family. And for that reason, your health is just as important as your family. Because without your health, you are likely going to have a hard time caring for, providing for, and being present for your family.

Ready for the next question?

▸ What is holding you back from exercising and getting in shape?

The most common response I get on this one? You probably guessed. It's some version of "lack of motivation."

But that isn't true. You don't lack motivation or willpower. I can prove it to you. Think about all the things that you do every single day that you aren't "motivated" to do. Get up when the alarm clock goes off. Take out the trash. Go to work when you'd rather go fishing or take a day off to watch Netflix. Keep your mouth shut instead of telling your bosses what you really think of them.

I ask the truck drivers, "Are you motivated to get up at two thirty a.m. and get paperwork signed or move the truck out of a dock? Are you motivated to drive thirty minutes out of route to go get the trailer washed out?" I give several examples of other annoying things that drivers hate doing but undertake nonetheless.

Once I can get them to agree that their health is of absolutely paramount importance in their world, I ask them this question:

Why is it that—when it comes your job—you do countless things whether you feel like it or not, whether you want to or not, whether you enjoy it or not? Yet, when it comes to what's most important in your life—your health—all of a sudden "how you feel" becomes the deciding factor?

It could be three in the morning and just ten degrees outside, and you will get up, get dressed, get out of the truck, and walk in your bills of lading. Yet you won't get up fifteen minutes earlier than scheduled to get in some quick but life-altering exercise? When the alarm clock goes off, you say to yourself, "I don't feel like getting up," so you don't?

I go through example after example of this contrast, pointing out the contradiction between their priorities and their behavior.

Then I explain to them the reason they behave this way. It is because of *consequences*. When it comes to their job, the consequences of not doing something are ever-present in their minds. Don't do something and they could damage their relationship with their fleet manager, who in turn won't give them the best loads, which will result in lost revenue. Don't do something and it could flat-out cost you your job. Then what will you do? How will you earn money? How will you pay rent and the bills and take care of your family? What if you end up homeless? Drivers—like most of us—will go to great measures to avoid these consequences, whether they like it or not.

Unfortunately, this isn't the case when it comes to promoting good health. The consequences are, unfortunately, not top of mind. We don't say to ourselves, *If I don't get up fifteen minutes earlier so that I can exercise, I will probably be the victim of metabolic syndrome and suffer one or more of the sixty medical disorders and twelve cancers, which will cost me my job, too.* We don't think that drinking the soda is going to force us to take diabetes medication. The consequences are more gradual and less direct. So we view them differently than we would the consequence of, say, showing up late to work.

When we have to get up for work, even if we don't feel like it, we do so because of the consequences. But when the moment comes to take action through exercise or choosing better food and drink options, the consequences of not doing so don't enter the equation. *That leaves room, then, for how we feel at that moment to dominate the decision-making process.* The further in the future the consequences are, the less influence they exert on our decision-making today. And, of course, we often don't feel like doing the "healthy" thing.

If you can do hundreds of things you hate doing without being motivated to do them, then you can exercise and make healthy food choices without being motivated to do them, either. The key is to educate yourself about the consequences of inaction. And then make this a priority. Just as important as writing down your goals is writing down the consequences of *not* changing your behavior.

That's why I developed the Goals Consequence Worksheet opposite: to help my clients understand both the opportunities ahead of them and the consequences of not taking advantage of those opportunities. Before your first workout, you will have completed the Fitness Goals Worksheet and made several copies of it. Read it every single day when you get up in the morning. Read it again before lunch. Before dinner. And before going to bed. In this way, you will train yourself to be conscious of your goals and consequences at strategic times when your actions have a maximum effect on your metabolism.

CONTROLLING YOUR
STRESS FOR OPTIMAL RESULTS

We think of truck drivers as free spirits. You see them on the interstate, sitting high in the saddle, maneuvering these enormous iron horses. And they are the Kings of the Road. But there is so much that is outside their control. A truck driver is a slave to his or her schedule, and drivers can't control their shifts or weather conditions or traffic on the road or an accident up ahead. They can't control shippers and receivers or when the freight arrives or the amount of paperwork required by the government. This combination of responsibility, uncertainty, and powerlessness causes a high degree of *stress*.

GOALS CONSEQUENCE WORKSHEET			
Goal	Action	Positive Consequence	Negative Consequence
Spike metabolism	4 minutes of vigorous activity	Maximum fat burning; weight loss; the body you want	No fat burning; metabolic syndrome; hospital; premature death; suboptimal life
Keep metabolism burning	Eat before starting your day, then eat every 3 hours	Maximum fat burning; weight loss; the body you want	No fat burning; metabolic syndrome; hospital; premature death; suboptimal life
Manage and reduce carbs	Log your food	Effective carb budgeting; metabolic efficiency; the body you want	Excess carbs and fat storage; metabolic syndrome; hospital; premature death; suboptimal life

Most of us can relate. Most of our jobs contain sources of stress. Stress comes in all sizes, and it comes at us from all angles. It might be different for a desk jockey who's facing a tight deadline than it is for a construction worker who has to brave the cold and work outdoors all day. Some jobs are dangerous; some lack security; some have tense interactions; some just simply don't pay enough to cover the bills.

Of course, there are also sources of stress outside of work. Financial pressures. Family pressures. Tough decisions. Sick family members. Put simply: stress is a fact of life. And *stress is a fundamental factor in the obesity crisis in America.* Fact is, *even if you eat healthily and exercise, high stress can hinder weight loss and even cause weight gain.* Put simply, stress = distress.

The body has a basic, evolutionary response to stress: we release a series of stress hormones, which trigger a fight-or-flight response. You either want to run away or want to punch somebody in the face. When this happens, there are several consequences. First, stress hormones cause fat cells throughout our bodies to release fatty acids into the bloodstream, so they can be used for fleeing or fighting. This was terrific when the stress was typically caused by charging lions or invading hordes, because we could use that energy to fight for survival. But when the stress is caused by a ticking clock and a traffic jam? Now you've got a lot of energy in the bloodstream and no way to burn it off.

So the hormone cortisol steps in, gathers up all those fatty acids, and stores them. Unfortunately, the easiest place for cortisol to store that fat is in our bellies. So the more stress we're under, the bigger our waistlines grow. Stress turns once-healthy peripheral fat into unhealthy visceral (or belly) fat in the abdomen. Visceral fat surrounds vital internal organs— primarily the liver—and releases harmful compounds that raise our cholesterol levels, damage our insulin sensitivity, and even raise our risk of some cancers. In fact, 60 percent of obese people have some degree of nonalcoholic fatty liver disease—basically, a cirrhosis-like scarring of the liver caused by visceral fat buildup. Nowadays, as many as 1 in 5 cases of liver failure is caused not by heavy drinking but by heaviness itself.

But the damage isn't over. Since our stores of energy have now been depleted (because they're on their way to our abdominal region), guess what happens? We get the signal that it's time to eat again. So we down more food (this is what's known as "stress eating") to quell those natural cravings. Of course, if you're in fight-or-flight mode, one of cortisol's functions is to shut down the top part of your brain, the cerebrum, where we do everything from memory storing to sensory processing to balancing our checkbook. In particular, it affects the frontal lobe, which—ordinarily—has the ability to override the impulse to make bad choices or engage in socially unacceptable behavior. Ever heard the expression "Don't make decisions while you're angry"? Well, there's something to it. Because when the brain is being flooded with cortisol, you literally can't think straight. You're being prevented from accessing the part of your brain necessary for making wise decisions. So now you're hungry, and your thinking is fuzzy, and you're probably being faced with a whole host of absolutely terrible food choices.

We see this all the time. When we're stressed, our internal circuits trip and our critical thinking powers shut down. In the case of trucking, I'll see a driver make a wrong turn. Then he panics, and the stress hormones kick in. What happens? He makes that second wrong turn and heads onto a bridge with low clearance or a single-lane road heading in the wrong direction. That's when drivers get into real trouble. It's not the first mistake that gets drivers into bad situations. It's the second mistake they make when they aren't thinking clearly and can't process the situation properly.

FIGHTING STRESS HEAD-ON

How do you handle the stress in your life? How do you change a stressful environment into a controlled one? The first step is to be aware of it and recognize the consequences. "I am experiencing stress, it's making me fat, and ultimately, it's shortening my life-span." Ask yourself: *Do I want to be doing this? Can I afford to keep living like this?* Assuming the answer is no, the question becomes: How am I going to deal with it?

Remember: knowledge is power, but *applied* knowledge is even more powerful. There are all sorts of methods for dealing with stress. Sometimes it just helps to take stock of the situation and think about the big picture.

In the case of truck drivers, it sometimes helps just to breathe, exhale, and then tell yourself—and you might even say it loudly in a calm tone—that ultimately it's no big deal. *There are factors beyond my control. If I'm going to be a little late, I'm going to be a little bit late. But I'm going to stay in the correct lane and continue to drive at a safe speed and not jeopardize my—or anyone else's—safety. I'll call the fleet manager, explain the situation, and they'll likely understand.* You are consciously calming yourself and reducing your stress. It all comes from awareness.

What else can you do more specifically? There are many ways to manage stress. At some level, it depends on the source. If it's financial, maybe it means sitting down and writing out a budget so you can start a savings plan. If it's related to marriage or relationships, maybe it means starting counseling. If it's related to general anxiety, maybe it's showing up for yoga sessions or meditating or practicing better sleep hygiene. Honestly, sex can—and should—be a part of a stress management program. For me, swim training is an effective way to deal with my stress. When I am in the water, I am relaxing mentally. When I finish with a swim practice, I feel accomplished and loosened up.

And—as with those four minutes of exercise—you have to force yourself, even if you're not motivated, even if you don't feel like it. Take your motivation (or lack of motivation) out of the equation. Just do it. Remember, you already have the skills you need every single day to override feelings of dread and to make yourself do things that might not be enjoyable but are necessary. You may not want to wake up early and go to work. But you do it anyway, because you know that, in the long run, it's important. *Can I pay my bills if I lose my job? No? Well, all right, I better get up even though I don't want to.*

We need to use those skills when we're dealing with something more important than our job: our health.

An analogy: It's the rare kid who likes brushing his teeth. I haven't met too many young kids who say, "You know what I love? The feeling of bristles on my tongue, the sensation of the bubbles on my tongue, and moving that toothbrush up and down against my gums. It's ecstasy." But parents require that kids brush their teeth. Then they get to a point where there's a risk-reward ratio. *I may not like brushing my teeth. But if I come to school with bad breath, I'll have a hard time getting a boyfriend or girlfriend.* Eventually it becomes a part of your routine, and you do it automatically, as a matter of habit, whether you feel like it or not.

The same thing applies here. One of the organizing principles of 4-Minute Fit: reach a point where you take motivation out of the equation. You decide that you're going to undertake a behavior—changing your diet, doing four minutes of vigorous exercise a day—whether you like it or not. Pretty soon, that behavior will harden into habit. Same goes for stress management.

Let's be clear: not all stress is bad stress. Living a life with no tension, never leaving your comfort zone, isn't entirely healthy, nor is it a way to achieve great things. These may sound like locker-room sports clichés, but stress is what makes us rise to challenges or overcome adversity. It's entirely possible to transfer bad stress ("I'm so angry at my boss") into something constructive ("I'll use that to exercise with greater intensity and get a greater metabolic effect"). Again, recognition is the key.

FAQ: I'm giving up smoking. Does that mean I'll gain weight?

I've never smoked cigarettes. Which means that I've never had to quit smoking. But I've seen firsthand how hard this can be. In addition to its many other health risks, nicotine is deeply addictive, which is to say that, even in the face of negative health consequences, people will compulsively seek out this drug. I respect anyone who quits smoking. I respect anyone who is *trying* to quit smoking.

It's hard enough to quit when you're determined, but it's even harder when you wind up talking yourself out of it. And here's one argument I've seen smokers use with themselves: *I don't want to quit smoking because I'll put on weight.* Put simply: it's just not true. Or it doesn't have to be true, anyway.

First, some facts. Yes, nicotine tends to boost the body's metabolism. (Immediately after you smoke a cigarette, your heart rate increases by 10 to 20 beats a minute.) This is unnatural and unhealthy—one reason smoking causes heart disease—but it's true that this increased heart rate may mean that your body temporarily increases the calories it burns. And if ex-smokers don't change their diets, they can pack on pounds. (But not much—studies show that even those former smokers who *do* put on weight put on an average of only five pounds.)

And, yes, there are researchers who claim that it's not just the nicotine that is addictive; it's the entire act of smoking. Just holding the cigarette in the fingers and bringing it up to your mouth can be a habit-forming behavior. When some people quit, they still seek to bring their hands to their mouths in a similar fashion, to recapture this oral gratification. And what do they do? They bring the hand to the mouth with food.

Another, similar school of thought goes like this: People smoke to relieve stress. They claim that smoking relaxes them. When they're not smoking, they feel anxious energy. If they don't satisfy this, they don't feel comfortable. (Although in truth, the only anxiety smoking alleviates is the anxiety caused by nicotine withdrawal.) So they interrupt this feeling of wanting something and satisfy it by eating. This is similar to emotional eating: There's a hole in your life—some comfort you're missing—and you're filling this void by eating. And soon you've reinforced this and you associate feeling better with eating. (And often eating the wrong foods.)

But you can take steps to avoid this.

I once had a driver explain to me how he quit smoking. He would take a handful of peanuts and would put one peanut in his mouth and chew it until it became a liquid. His doing this mimicked smoking. He got the hand-to-mouth sensation. It took roughly the same time to eat the peanuts as it took to smoke a cigarette. Fortunately, peanuts are mostly protein and healthy, monounsaturated fat, and contain very few carbs, so even though this driver was eating (almost constantly!), this was good for his metabolism. And fortunately, he was doing something to satisfy his neuromuscular activity requirement. *Hey, I should be doing something with my hand and my mouth.* So this was an intelligent substitution.

Here are other edible alternatives to smoking that provide the oral gratification:

Sugar-free candy

Slivers of vegetables like celery stalks or carrot sticks

There are other ways to get the oral gratification beyond consuming food. You can chew gum. You can also brush your teeth throughout the day. (Having fresh breath and a feeling of oral hygiene reduces the urge to smoke.)

Another solution is activity. Just staying busy is a way to distract yourself from smoking. Go out with a friend. Go to the movies or a concert, where smoking is almost always banned anyway. If you go on a bike ride or play sports or go for a walk, you have the added bonus of burning calories. I've had clients tell me that they were so busy they didn't have time to remember they were missing cigarettes.

Of course, there are smoking-cessation programs, too, that use drugs to help you quit. Though my experience is that people in these programs don't necessarily plan to reduce and eliminate nicotine consumption; they go from smoking to vaporizing/e-cigarette use because they believe it's preferable, which it may well be. But they have no real plan to quit.

Bottom line: there doesn't need to be a cause-and-effect relationship here. The key question: how are you replacing the smoking? Have a strategy!

People who smoke are short of breath and resistant to exertion. Quit smoking, and you'll feel far more comfortable with starting an exercise routine. In almost every case, swapping cigs for sweat will result in weight loss—and save you hundreds, maybe thousands of dollars a year in health-care costs, not to mention the cost of a carton every week.

8 Nutrition Secrets for Rapid Weight Loss

When it comes to nutrition, *everything you have been taught is wrong.*

Most of us have been brought up to believe that there are certain immutable laws of nutrition. Never mind that those laws seem to change every few years: low-fat, full-fat, vegan, Paleo—having strict rules makes us feel like we have control. But that control is an illusion.

The first thing I always tell drivers: *nutrition is dynamic.* This means nutrition is a vital and changing process, dependent on your state and circumstance. What works for you at one phase of your life may not work for you in another. What works for you when you live in one climate may not work for you when you move to another. What works for you in one job may not work for you in another.

What this also means is that there is no one diet that everyone should follow, no one-size-fits-all method to lose weight and lead a healthier life. *Everyone should eat Paleo! Everyone should be a vegetarian! Or everyone should eat Mediterranean.* Sorry, it doesn't work like that. To find the nutrition plan that works for your body, you need to start with an open mind.

WHY WE CAN'T (AND SHOULDN'T!) STICK TO A DIET

After I had left Yale and started exploring the world, I started coming into contact with new people, new theories, and new ideas. A lot of those ideas centered on health and nutrition.

I met an African doctor who was working in Chicago, and I explained to him that I had suffered from sinus problems from as early as I could remember. When I was a kid, we called it "hay fever." Like clockwork, it would come on in late August as the summer wound to a close, and by September I was a congested mess, sniffling and going nowhere without Kleenexes—snot rags, we called them—stuffed in my pockets. At night, I was even more miserable. I couldn't breathe out of my nose, and the only thing I could do to get to sleep was to go for a pre-bed (or middle-of-the-night) run around the block, because that was the only way that my sinuses would clear up. I would have ten minutes of clear breathing, and I would have to fall asleep during that interval. Otherwise, it would be a long, sleepless night.

Anyway, the doctor was quick to diagnose the problem. "You don't have hay fever or allergies to pollen," he said with self-assurance.

I don't?

"No," he explained. "You have what is called catarrhal condition. Catarrh is a term that means internal inflammation. You're poisoning yourself from the inside out. Stop eating meat, yeast, and dairy products. Those products are fermenting in your belly and producing a gas. And that gas is irritating your mucus membranes. You're already irritated and then, when you come into contact with particles or pollen in the environment, your body can't handle it. The root of your condition is in your gut!"

I shrugged and decided to try his advice. I cut out meat, yeast, and dairy from my diet. And I started to get better. August and the fall would come and go, and I wasn't sniffling or having to do heavy exercise just to get to sleep.

A few years after that, when I joined the Rasta movement, I was introduced to their diet, which is very strict. No meat, no animal products, no processed food. That started me on a path to being a vegetarian and a vegan for fifteen years. I was eating whole grains, fresh fruits and vegetables, and tofu. I stayed away from processed foods like chips and canned vegetables. And my girlfriend at the time enjoyed cooking, so I wasn't just eating salad. She would spend significant amounts of time preparing gourmet vegetarian meals. I was convinced that I was practicing the healthiest diet on the planet.

Then, in my late thirties, I got into trucking. I was still a vegetarian, but suddenly I was not eating the kinds of vegetarian meals I was used to. I was not exercising as much as I used to. I was gaining weight. And something happened that I wasn't used to: I starting to get sick, something that had rarely happened to me before that.

I thought I had an idea why. As I was doing so much driving around, my environment was changing. I was going from, say, a hot and humid climate in Georgia one day, to a colder climate in Chicago the next day. Then I would go out west, and the weather would be different. My habits were starting to slip. I was still sticking to a vegetarian diet, but when you're on the road, "vegetarian" tends to look like French fries and nachos instead of fresh fruits and vegetables. And I kept getting sick.

Finally, I realized that I had to make a choice: either I was going to stay a vegetarian or I was going to get healthy. It became clear that the very diet that had helped me at one point in my life was now hurting me. I went back to eating meat. And soon I was getting results.

Now fast-forward a few years. I am going through a divorce, and it is causing me great anxiety. For a few months, I am suffering from insomnia. I am feeling fatigued and exhausted and generally lousy.

I consulted a specialist in Eastern medicine. He performed what he called a "pulse diagnostic" on me, essentially a diagnosis based on the five-organ method of traditional Chinese medicine. He said, "Listen, Siphiwe, your spleen energy system—the system responsible from extracting energy from food—is completely depleted. So much so that it doesn't matter how good a diet you've adopted or how nutritious the food you eat is, your body is not extracting the nutrition from it. All that organic, grass-fed beef or fresh fruit? You're not getting the benefit. In fact, I want you to stay away from uncooked fruits and vegetables."

Wait, what? You're telling me to stay away from raw fruits and vegetables, supposedly the healthiest food you can eat?

He explained that when you eat raw fruits and vegetables, your body first has to heat up the food to 100 degrees before you can digest it. In fact, the nutrients in many foods, especially vegetables, become more "bioavailable" when we cook them. "For a system already taxed like yours is, when you eat raw fruits and vegetables, it's harder for your body to digest it. You need to cook everything, eat lots of stews. When you cook food, you actually predigest it and make it easier on your body. You might destroy some of the nutrition in the cooking, but your body will able to absorb more of it."

So here's the point: different junctures of my life have required different diets.

THE MYTH OF "JUNK" FOOD

As I mentioned in an earlier chapter, when I first starting working with truck drivers, I assumed that so many of them are overweight because of overeating.

But when I started looking at the data, it turned out that wasn't the case at all. What I found: drivers—like most obese people—aren't glutonous. Most of them are undereating, consuming fewer than three meals a day, more like 2.6 on average. Many skipped breakfast, but some of them skipped lunch and/or dinner. Most people with a busy lifestyle do this, too. We eat twice a day and don't think much of it. (In fact, we probably assume it's good for us.)

And not only were the truckers I studied burning more calories than they were consuming, a lot of the time their bodies were in starvation mode. How could this be? Well, they weren't eating frequently enough, which means they weren't giving their metabolism any work to do during the day. Their metabolism had been turned down to the lowest level.

I'll talk more about metabolism in an upcoming chapter, but the fact is that the efficiency of our metabolism determines how much energy we extract from our food and how much energy we have to get through the day. When we're extracting energy and making it available, our metabolisms run high, and we burn off fat. When we don't, no amount of food restriction and self-denial is going to take off the weight.

That's why it's so important not to get caught up in lists of foods we "can't ever eat" or alternatively, "superfoods" we have to eat every day. I understand why we like quick-and-easy lists. They simplify concepts and help us make priorities. As anyone who's taken even a casual glance at the Internet these days will tell you, when it comes to diet and nutrition, you can find all sorts of lists: "Ten Ways to Lose Weight," "Five Ways to Tighter Abs," "Ten Best Burritos for Your Biceps." These lists are usually ridiculous oversimplifications. One in particular kind of list that always gets me: "Five Foods to Avoid at All Costs."

Here's the truth: nothing in the universe works that way. As any *Star Wars* fan can tell you, nothing—and no person or thing—is entirely good or entirely bad. With nutrition, it works the same way. Some foods might be better than others. But none is entirely good or bad. For example, a plain white baguette has a glycemic index of 95. That's extremely high. That means that the baguette will quickly raise blood sugar. For most of us, that's a prescription for weight gain. And for someone who already has high blood sugar, eating the baguette will spike the blood sugar even higher. This can lead to hyperglycemia. (If you have type 2 diabetes or if you're at risk for it, extremely high blood sugar can even lead to a potentially deadly condition in which your body can't process sugar. It's called *hyperosmolar hyperglycemic nonketotic syndrome*, HHNS.)

For others, that baguette can come in handy as a fitness and weight-loss tool. To use myself as an example, when I was training for the 2012 Ironman South Africa, I would have these long training days that started at 4:30 in the morning. I would ride more than a hundred miles on my bike, then run ten miles. I was in constant need of glucose in my system to prevent the massive fatigue known as "bonking." In such a case, eating a baguette would very quickly give me the glucose I needed. Again, the point is to illustrate that everything is relative. In this plan, there is nothing that is absolutely forbidden.

That said, some foods are better than others, or, stated more precisely, some foods have *greater nutritive value* than others. And for people who are battling diabetes or simply want to lose significant amounts of weight, there are some foods that really work against these goals—in particular, foods that have lots of carbs and little nutritional value. If weight loss is my goal, here are the foods I would definitely avoid:

1. **Any drink with calories or carbs:** sodas, fruit juices, sweet teas, and energy drinks. Because liquid calories are ab-

sorbed more quickly than food calories, they overwhelm the body's ability to burn them off; we have no choice but to turn liquid calories into fat, fast. You can think of any high-calorie drink as delivering fat right to your gut.

2. **Rice:** doesn't matter if it's white, brown, basmati, or jasmine. Because it's usually low in fiber and protein but high in carbs, rice adds plenty of unnecessary calories with little nutritional impact.

3. **Bread:** doesn't matter if it's white, whole wheat, multi-grain, flatbread, wrap, et cetera. Even wheat breads are carbohydrate-delivery systems with little nutritional value.

4. **French fries:** Most of the nutrients and fiber in potatoes are found in the skin. But with fries, we peel off the nutrition, then douse the taters in oil and salt. As a result, we get plenty of sodium, carbs, and fat but little that's of use to our bodies.

5. **Pasta:** especially if it's served with heavy sauces and garlic bread!

But while the above points are good guidelines, you can't follow them all the time. You can't constantly eat the same food, over and over. You also can't continually deprive yourself of the enjoyment of eating food.

In the case of drivers, 90 percent of them eat at the spots alongside the interstate. That means truck stops and the fast-food outlets inside. That also means Denny's and Ruby Tuesday and Olive Garden and Country Buffet and Red Lobster. Some of this is practical. You're driving in parts of the country where you don't always have a huge choice of restaurants. You're usually driving a 53-foot steel whale, and you're not able to drive into town and find the precious restaurant with quinoa and grass-fed beef. (And if you do find it, you're not exactly guaranteed a place to park!)

But more than that, drivers *like* these chain restaurants. They tell me that there is a feeling of familiarity—you know what you're getting. The food tastes the same, looks the same, smells the same, even feels the same in the packaging and in their hands. They say that the portions are generous, and the food tastes good. Instead of trying to convince them otherwise, I have two simple messages:

1. I'm not going to require you to change your routine radically, because that's unsustainable and it's overwhelming. You will likely fail at your diet if you try to make a big change like that. I'm not going to tell you to eat at different restaurants. What I *am* going to tell you: *log your nutrition.*

2. Tied to that, use the tools at your disposal and make change you are comfortable with making. Read the nutritional information, look at the calorie count, and make the informed choice. If you really want the chicken-fried steak over the grilled chicken, the plan won't stop you. But realize the consequences. If you can switch to a burrito bowl (without the tortilla) instead of the regular burrito you're used to eating, realize that will have consequences, too—positive ones.

HOW TO USE FOOD TO SPIKE YOUR METABOLISM

In chapter 9, you'll read more about the process of metabolism, and
why your metabolism has the final say in whether you'll lose weight
or gain it. But there are three rules of eating that are critical to keeping
your metabolism running hot.

1. Eat Breakfast and Then Eat Something Every Three Hours

When I began implementing 4-Minute Fit, I started with the usual assumption: my job would consist primarily of teaching drivers how to
cut back on the food they ate. I thought I would be using their food
logs to show them ways to reduce their calorie intake. To my great
surprise, however, I discovered something entirely different.

Of the first fifty drivers I worked with, *none*—not a one!—of them
had a calorie surplus. All of them actually had a calorie deficit: The average calories burned in the first week of the program was 3,575. The
actual calorie consumption was just 1,539 calories.

What?

To my surprise, most of the drivers were eating only once or twice a day. They may have been overeating at either or both of those meals, but their nutrition for the entire day or week was actually insufficient. I realized that the vast majority of drivers were skipping meals. As a result, they were going long periods without eating anything—and without giving their metabolism any work to do.

According to Dr. John Berardi, a nutritionist I really admire:

> *Although you might think that eating less would help prevent weight gain, it actually slows your metabolism ... [M]odern-day humans have a quite sensitive mechanism that fairly quickly turns down metabolism when it senses that fewer calories are coming in. When you go too many hours without eating or dramatically reduce your overall calorie intake, your brain tells the cells in your body to slow down the works, and you burn fewer overall calories as a result. Your body also starts to burn carbohydrates and muscle protein for energy, preserving your fat. Less muscle equals a prematurely lowered RME [resting metabolic expenditure].*
>
> *Restricting calories slows metabolism for yet another, lesser known reason. It reduces your overall metabolic flux—the flow of energy into and out of your body. Energy flows into the metabolic systems of your body when you eat, and it flows out of them when you burn calories (through planned exercise and daily movement) ... When you put more energy into the system (by eating more) and take more energy out of the system (by exercising more), you increase your flux. Consequently, your metabolism must work harder to process all of those calories. The higher your flux, the higher your metabolism*

This goes a long way to explain why the drivers were obese and had so much fat. The problem wasn't that they were overeating; the problem was that they had very little flux. They were skipping meals—not putting energy into the system—and they were sedentary as many as twenty-three hours a day (not taking energy out of the system). So their overall metabolic flux was extremely low. *To counsel these drivers with the old "eat less" advice was to do more damage.* What these drivers needed to do was to eat more, and specifically, eat more frequently. The drivers needed to give their metabolism work to do while they were driving, and that meant eating every three hours. More specifically, it meant eating the right foods every three hours.

What are the right foods? Since it is carbohydrates that get converted to glucose and eventually get stored as fat in sedentary people, obese people will want to limit their carbohydrate consumption. This includes "good" and "bad," "simple" and "complex" carbs. Carbs are carbs. It doesn't matter if they are simple or complex; if your body doesn't need the energy, they both get stored as fat.

Protein, on the other hand, is different. Proteins are the body's building blocks. When you build things to last, you build them out of strong material. You don't want the big bad wolf to come huff and puff and blow your house down, so instead of building with weak materials like straw, you build with strong materials like wood, brick, or stone. Compared to carbohydrates, proteins are strong materials. Your body burns twice as many calories to digest high-protein foods as it does for high-carb foods. That means your metabolism has to work longer and harder to digest protein. Since the purpose of eating in 4-Minute Fit is to *drive metabolism* in obese, sedentary people, eating the right foods means eating foods high in protein and low in carbs. This should be done every three hours.

For people whose schedules change frequently or who work the night shift, eating every three hours can be challenging. These circumstances have a disrupting effect on circadian rhythms, which also affects hormone production. This can prevent the body from regulating hunger properly. You may not feel hungry because the hormone that stimulates appetite isn't being produced properly. Nevertheless, in 4-Minute Fit, it is important to eat every three hours whether you feel hungry or not. It doesn't have to be a full-blown meal. A handful of almonds, a low-fat cheese stick, some tuna are all good examples of between-meal snacks.

Whether you are behind the wheel or behind a computer, behind a desk, behind a bar, working at a factory or hospital, sedentary or active, if your goal is to burn fat, then you need to eat breakfast—to start your metabolism at the beginning of the day (or at the beginning of your shift) —and then eat every three hours.

2. Always Eat After a Workout

Eating food—particularly carbohydrates—does less damage to weight-loss efforts when it's done after a workout. Why? Because the increased metabolic demand post-workout is much higher than normal, so your body is primed to torch any carbohydrates you eat, rather than convert them to fat storage. In other words, if you eat a banana while driving or sitting at your desk, your body doesn't need the energy. So most of the 27 grams of carbohydrates in the banana will get converted to fat and stored in the body.

But if you eat that same banana right after a workout, when there is a very high demand for energy, many of the carbohydrates consumed will be used in the metabolic processes and *not* converted to fat and stored in the body. As a result, there is a "best time" to eat some of your favorite foods that contain a lot of simple carbohydrates. Eating them after a workout will do less damage. Knowing this can make it easier to adhere to the program. You'll learn that you don't have to deprive yourself all the time.

In addition, eating right after a workout helps the body recover by replenishing electrolytes, amino acids, and other nutrients. The sooner and the more thoroughly you recover from a workout, the less sore and sluggish you'll be. Also, the fewer aftereffects you feel, the more likely you will be to exercise the next day.

If you're interested, there are even more complex mechanisms at work here, too. Here is how it is explained in the book *Nutrient Timing System*:

> *The Anabolic Phase is the forty-five-minute window following a workout in which your muscle machinery, in the presence of the right combination of nutrients, initiates the repair of damaged muscle protein and replenishes muscle glycogen stores. Immediately after exercise, muscle cells are extremely sensitive to the anabolic effects of the hormone insulin ... Nutrients consumed during this post-exercise "metabolic window" are much more effective than those consumed later, when the muscle becomes insulin resistant ... Consuming high-glycemic carbohydrates following exercise stimulates insulin ... When insulin is stimulated in the presence of protein, the result is greater synthesis of new protein. In other words, carbohydrates prime the protein pump by first stimulating insulin. A complex carbohydrate is less effective because it is a weaker stimulator of insulin.*

But here's what's most important to understand: just about anything eaten after a workout is going to have beneficial effects. Eating something after a workout—even a doughnut!—is going to be better than eating nothing at all. Is a Snickers bar a great idea for a snack? Maybe. It depends. But if you love Snickers, is there a best time to eat one? You bet. Right after a workout! Consider it your reward for a job well done. Just not every day.

3. Keep Healthy Snacks Within Reach

Here's a way to: (a) eat every three hours after breakfast and (b) remember to eat after working out: keep healthy snacks within reach. For my drivers, this meant stopping at a grocery store once a week to buy snacks they would keep on the truck. For others, this may mean bringing the right meals and snack to the office and keeping them in your desk. For others, it's leaving snacks in your locker. The old Boy Scout motto applies: "Be prepared!"

If you don't keep healthy snacks within reach, then one of two scenes is likely to unfold: either you have unhealthy snacks within reach, or you have no snacks within reach. Not eating, as I hope I've drilled into you by now, can be just as bad as eating the wrong thing!

HOW TO MANAGE YOUR HUNGER

I get this question a lot, and anyone who's ever dieted can probably relate to this:

I'm doing great and feeling in control. I'm committed to following my plan this day. A few hours go by and everything is going great. Then hunger hits and my willpower evaporates. Suddenly, I just want to eat. I mean EAT. Like, anything in sight. And these few minutes of weakness disrupt everything and set me back. What can I do to stop this?

While most overweight people are actually malnourished, there's no doubt that bouts of intense hunger can creep up on us just when we're starting to achieve some success with our weight-loss plan.

There's no simple answer to the question of hunger pangs, but here's a start: understand what's actually going on in your body and mind. First, how do we know when we're hungry? It comes mostly from the brain, not the belly. It's not because our stomach growls. (There are people who have had their stomach removed who still feel hunger.) A part of the brain called the hypothalamus is the center of hunger, sensing when we need to eat.

The feeling of hunger is regulated by metabolism. Your body secretes hormones that circulate in the blood. These hormones communicate with a neurotransmitter called NPY that send messages to the brain: *Hey, I need nourishment.* Ghrelin is a hormone that stimulates your appetite. Leptin is a hormone, made by fat cells, that decreases your appetite and tells you that you're full or no longer hungry. A person whose metabolism is functioning properly is producing these hormones in the right proportions and at the right times.

The greatest portion of these hormones is produced in our sleep. When we suffer sleep deprivation, it throws our hunger hormones out of whack. Therefore, the first step to getting in control of hunger is getting optimal sleep.

So after a few hours without anything to eat, ghrelin and the NPY neurotransmitter activate, and you feel hungry? Great. That's normal—especially if you've been active, exercising, or engaged in other activity that stimulates your ghrelin. You want to eat, and you should eat. The key, of course, is training your body to eat the right things. Typically, when we feel really hungry, we eat the wrong foods.

In part, this is biological. According to at least one theory, low levels of glycogen and low blood sugar levels stimulate a spike in ghrelin and NPY activity in the hypothalamus. As the hypothalamus is stimulated, our desire for sweet and starchy foods goes up. Skipping meals increases the NPY levels, setting us up for a carbohydrate binge. Worse, when we indulge in junk food, the brain sends signals telling us that our bodies haven't gotten the nutrition we were seeking. And so, guess what? We need to eat more. So we're not only eating the wrong foods, but eating too much of them.

But it's also because we've trained our bodies to *want* the wrong foods. When we sense hunger coming on, we're trained to react to it immediately with foods that are easy to prepare. This often means processed foods and foods with little nutritional value. This becomes habit: *Hey, it's snack time, that means chips.* Unwrap and eat. And repeat.

What should we eat, especially at times of intense hunger? Lean protein that will give your metabolism work to do. Fiber that will make you feel full. But this is also why nutritional supplements can be so important. When you feed the body this concentrated nutrition via these supplements, you're getting most of what you need, and so the brain is not signaling the body to eat more. If the nutrition is already in you, you've gone a long way toward solving the I-want-to-eat-everything level of hunger.

Also, a lot of times hunger is situational and conditioned behavior. It's what we call "emotional eating." Here's an example from the trucking world that happens to a lot of drivers including me: I'd eat breakfast and then I'd be driving for a few hours. By midmorning I'd be fighting driver fatigue and boredom. So I would eat because I was bored, not hungry. Midafternoon, same thing. I was hungry for something. But it wasn't necessarily food. It was just stimulation I craved, but my brain confused it with hunger. I filled the emotional need, this discomfort, with food. I ate food—usually the sweet and salty kind—to stimulate the pleasure center in the brain. If I had recognized and identified this, and kept emotional hunger separate from physical hunger, I would have tried to fill this need with another kind of pleasure.

Remember: *hunger is natural.* It's the body's way of telling ourselves we need nourishment. It's what we eat when we're hungry that matters. Knowing your body and knowing yourself will help you make the right choices when hunger strikes.

The Hunger Game

But I haven't really answered the question, What do I do when I feel this intense craving? So here's what you do:

1. Ask yourself, have I eaten in the last three hours? If no, then make the decision to eat.
2. If yes, then ask yourself, did I eat mostly carbs or mostly protein? If it was mostly carbs, then eat a small protein snack with little to no carbs such as a handful of almonds or a low-fat cheese stick.
3. If you ate mostly protein, you can eat a snack with protein and a little more carbs, but pay attention to your carb budget.
4. Immediately occupy yourself with something you are very interested in and excited about. Surf the Internet; grab your book or magazine and read a quick article. Or practice visualizing some goal or future event.

The idea is to switch your mind and attention from the food craving (after having fed yourself something) and to something that excites you. When you are focused and engaged in something, feeding yourself inspiration, you become less aware that you are hungry. Mentally, you feel satisfied. And that triggers a biochemical change.

FAQ: I'm traveling, and that's usually when I fall off my nutrition plan. What can I do to stick to it?

There's no reason to blow up your diet or fitness plan because you're away from home. *I'm on the road, so there's a substantial change?* Not so. (Remember, this is a program that originally was designed for people who spend three hundred or so days and nights on the road!) If anything, it's that mentality that needs to change. As usual, it all comes down to planning.

▸ Pack some supps. Remember, I recommend that as a foundation of your nutrition you use concentrated nutrition supplements. Look for versions that come in individual packets, such as the IsaLean Pro shake. It's easy, it's convenient, it provides 75 percent of the nutrition you need for the entire day. You open the packet, combine it with some water, shake it up, and drink it. Adopt that as a strategy, and all you need to do is bring the supplements with you. Gone for five days? Bring five packs. Simple. Regardless of what's available at the hotel, whether you get a continental breakfast or not, you're starting the day as you did at home.

▸ Go easy on lunch. Unpredictability is often an unavoidable part of business travel. If you have a light, low-carb lunch, you have a big food budget left over for dinner. Even if the boss says, "Come with us, I made a reservation at the local steakhouse," or even if you are done with your meetings late and all that's available is room service, you can eat (relatively) freely.

▶ If you are tracking your food and have a "carb budget," then when you're eating out, you're employing the same principles as you do at home. What can I afford to eat? Can I eat hamburger with a big bun that has a lot of carbs? Can I eat fries? Pizza? Beer? Probably not. Then again, you can substitute. (Want that burger for lunch? Maybe you can have it, if you are willing to eat extra healthy at dinner.) And you can modify. Want that chicken sandwich? Maybe you get it without the bun or without the mayo or with the vegetable or salad instead of the side of fries. Again, do what you would do at home: look at your options and make the best available choice.

▶ Pack your snacks. You packed a suitcase, a carry-on bag, and a toiletry kit, right? Well, pack some healthy snacks as well. If you're not eating at regular intervals on the road, you can make sure you're not skipping meals entirely by digging into snacks. Almonds, pumpkin seeds, low-fat cheese sticks, tuna, and Nature Valley Protein Chewy bars are all good choices. Having an array of snacks handy will ensure your metabolism keeps chugging along.

▶ Drink lots of water. Yes, it's the fallback you hear all the time—the dieting equivalent to "dress in layers"—but that doesn't mean that it's wrong. In truth, drinking water will help everything from reducing jet lag to flushing the body of toxins. Studies also show that water will reduce cravings.

FAQ: Does sex count as my four minutes?

I'll avoid making a wisecrack about four minutes and simply point out that as much as we all enjoy sex (and as hard as we're sometimes breathing during and after), it is not prime exercise. According to one study, your average romp between married partners burns fewer than 50 calories. This is the equivalent of a leisurely walk around the block or a walk up just two flights of stairs. Sorry.

WHY EATING HEALTHY IS CHEAPER

Here are two riffs I overhear at work that make me stop what I'm doing and react:

- ▶ "I'm eating like crap, but at least these Value Meals are cheap."

- ▶ "I want to eat healthier, but I can't afford it; those thirteen-dollar lunches from the Whole Foods salad bar are way out of my price range."

In the first scenario—the person who thinks he's getting a better economic deal for eating like crap—we see a person who's making a terrible long-term investment. Study after study shows how costly it is to be obese, both for the individual and for society. And it doesn't stop there. Obese people are less likely to be hired, less likely to be promoted, and less likely to get raises; plus, they incur hidden costs, like putting extra gas into their cars to accommodate their extra weight.

We're talking about thousands—perhaps tens of thousands—of

dollars a year taken from your paychecks and personal income just for being obese. That's a lot of Value Meals! Let's be clear: living an unhealthy life comes with a lot of hidden costs.

What's more, eating healthy doesn't necessarily mean eating $13 lunches at Whole Foods. One personal example: right now I am a single father with shared custody. I have a busy life, and I try to get the "busy" out of the way before my boys come to me on weekends. One way I try to maximize time is to do the meal preparation before they arrive—without losing and destroying the nutrients from the food. So several times a week, I'll buy some celery, carrots, onions, and garlic at the local organic market, and a whole organic free-range chicken. (It costs a little more, but not dramatically more, and the nutritional payoff of local, organic food is worth it.) I'll chop up the vegetables, dump everything into a Crock-Pot, throw in some seasonings, and slow-cook this.

Start to finish, it might take me twenty minutes to prepare, and then the slow cooker does the rest. We're talking basic ingredients. (Other favorites of mine: beets, okra, spinach—nothing exotic—with some sort of meat.) It might cost $20, tops. And this will feed three of us for dinner and lunch the next day—with some left over. We're talking six to eight healthy, organic meals from one food prep, for maybe $20. That's no $13 salad! (In fact, it's a lot less expensive than those "value meals" at the chicken joint.)

There are infinite combinations for eating healthy. There are also countless substitutions—for both your personal taste preferences and your finances. Don't want to buy a whole organic chicken? Use fish, turkey, bison, or lean beef. Don't want to eat pasta? Try spaghetti squash; it's an inexpensive base that mimics pasta, without all the carbs. Spaghetti squash with tomato sauce and some chicken, shrimp, or bison sausage? That's tasty and supremely nutritious. And it's costing you much less than dinner at Chili's or Applebee's.

In my experience, people who worry about the cost of healthy just need to change their concept of eating healthy. It doesn't have to mean fancy gourmet preparation, and it doesn't have to mean dropping big money at Whole Foods. (Or, as even President Obama once joked, Whole Paycheck.) No, learn how to prepare some of the many meals that are time-effective and tasty. Don't overcook the food, which causes a loss of nutrients. And you know what you get? A *real* Value Meal!

FAQ: Is a protein bar a good substitute for a meal?

No! Protein bars may pack a lot of nutrition, but they're not the same as eating a proper meal. For one, they are highly processed, and processed food usually requires fewer calories to digest. Second, "protein bars" is a hugely broad food category. Some of them (starting with the homemade variety) are thoroughly healthy and perfectly tasty. Others are fancied-up candy bars, filled with ingredients like corn syrup and chocolate. The convenience of protein bars cannot be denied. They're easy to acquire, easy to eat, fast, and low-maintenance. But think of them as snacks. And do so only after reading the ingredients carefully. Generally speaking, it's better to get your nutrition from real food than from supplements like protein shakes and protein bars. Nevertheless, they can be very helpful. The best way to find out where such items fit into your nutrition plan is to establish your nutrition profile first, determine your protein consumption, and identify if and when you are not getting enough quality protein. With the help of the nutrition logging apps I keep talking about, it's a very easy process.

MAKE YOUR WORKPLACE WORK FOR YOU

Part of the appeal of driving a truck is the unpredictability. One day you're in the mountains, the next day you're driving through the prairie. One week you'll drive through Maine with the heat cranked up. The next week you'll be driving in Arizona with the A/C blasting. When people say "No two days are ever alike," it definitely applies to this line of work.

One of the drawbacks of driving, though, is that it's hard to plan your diet. Even with apps and digital technology, it can be hard to know when (and whether) you'll come across a suitable restaurant. You don't always know what truck stop you'll have or what options will be available there. You don't know when traffic or bad road conditions will disrupt your schedule.

People with more conventional office jobs—and more predictability—are in a better position to plan their meals and snacks. But the office workplace is still filled with traps. Here are three tips for sticking to your diet in the office:

> ▶ Get up from your workstation. Eating at your desk might be a way to show your superiors how committed and busy you are. And it might be a way to bang out some emails or stay on a conference call, multitasking that helps your efficiency. (And might enable you to leave work a little early.) But it can be bad for your diet. According to a study in the *American Journal of Clinical Nutrition*, workers who ate their lunch while playing a computer game ended up eating more cookies thirty minutes later than those who hadn't been gaming. That's what's known as "distracted eating," and it's exactly the opposite of what you need to be doing: keeping track of what

you eat and being mindful of your carb intake. Staring at a screen while you eat is a guaranteed way to lose focus on what you're putting into your mouth.

▶ You're better off trying to make some time—even if it's a few minutes—to eat in the cafeteria or conference room or break room. Better yet, go outdoors to eat.

▶ So carve out twenty minutes a day (we know, you've got a million things to do, but . . .) and eat in your conference room or break room (or outdoors!). Multiple studies show that eating outdoors or in an environment where you can be "engaged effortlessly" helps the brain refresh and can be a trigger for creativity.

▶ Turn a colleague into a coach. Workplace gossip is as much a part of most offices as copier jams and email outages at the worst times possible. Some workers indulge more than others. But if you can gently ask around and find out who else might be trying to improve their diet and fitness, it could really benefit you. Having a colleague with fitness goals close to yours might provide you with a kindred spirit. You might snack together, plan your lunches together, or simply be there for each other when cravings hit or when the willpower lapses.

FAQ: Does microwaving zap nutrients?

For many of us, as we get busier and busier—and our time more valuable, and therefore sacred, than ever—the microwave oven has become one of the most important appliances in our lives. It's easy to feel ambivalent about this and be nostalgic for the days when we used to cook with grills and conventional ovens, and we had more than forty-five seconds to get our food warm. But this is a cultural problem, not a nutritional problem. The heat and length of time affects nutrition, but not the cooking method. Cooking for a long time or at a high heat affects water content and certain heat-sensitive nutrients, such as thiamine. Some researchers even believe that because microwave ovens cook food so quickly, they can actually help to minimize the loss of nutrients. The jury is still out on this. My personal preference is to avoid the microwave as a way of cooking meals, but I don't freak out if I am in a situation and the microwave is all that I have, especially if I am just reheating leftovers.

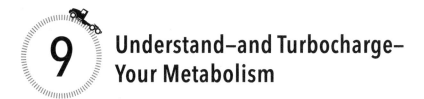

9 Understand–and Turbocharge–Your Metabolism

THE SECRET TO KEEPING YOUR FAT BURNERS AT MAXIMUM CAPACITY

Throughout the first few chapters of this book, you've been reading an awful lot about metabolism. You've seen how trying to burn off fat and calories through exercise simply doesn't work; how trying to lose weight by skipping meals doesn't work either; and how using a combination of brief, metabolism-spiking workouts and regular meals throughout the day will set you up for twenty-four-hour fat burning, no matter how sedentary your life may be.

But "metabolism" is still a little bit of a fuzzy concept. So in this chapter, I want to focus on exactly how it works and why our typical American lifestyle is slowing our metabolisms down in ways we might never have expected.

Metabolism is a complicated concept, but here's how I like to simplify it: *metabolism is the process for producing energy in the body.*

People who are obese, who are sedentary, whose work schedules interfere with their circadian rhythms and sleep schedules, or who are under a lot of stress, all face the same issue: *they have inefficient me-*

tabolisms. All of this is totally understandable for reasons I'll explain below. But if you fall into this category, the immediate goal should be making your metabolism more efficient and more effective.

How do we do that? Well, let's start at the cellular level. Energy is produced in a specific place inside of every cell, the mitochondria. And in order to produce energy, the mitochondria need what's called *adenosine triphosphate* (ATP) for fuel. The more mitochondria you have and the bigger the mitochondria you have, the more potential capacity you have to produce energy, and the higher your overall metabolism (and daily calorie burn) will be. Think of mitochondria as the burners on your grill: the more you have, and the higher they're cranked up, the more energy you'll burn off every single minute of the day.

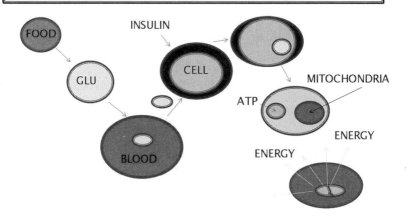

ENERGY PRODUCTION

So 4-Minute Fit is designed to address the issues that inhibit the production of ATP, causing us to create energy inefficiently and hence become slower, fatter, hungrier, and more tired. Our goal is to muscle up your mitochondria! Here's how we do it.

BETTER METABOLISM THROUGH SLEEP

Your metabolism and energy cycles are controlled by a complex series of hormones. Again, I like to describe hormones as signals in the body that stimulate processes and get us to act. You haven't eaten in a while? Your body will send you signals saying that you need some raw materials (i.e., food) to produce fuel. That's a signal from the "hunger hormone" ghrelin, which is produced in your sleep. The hormone is secreted, it triggers you to eat, and that's the way to ensure that you have the raw materials for energy production. When your ghrelin is high, we get hungry and crave "unhealthy" foods. When your ghrelin is low, hunger decreases. Meanwhile, the hormone leptin regulates the signal that tells you to stop eating. What happens when you go to fill up your car or truck with gas, you leave the gas pump nozzle in the fuel tank, and you put it on automatic? If there's no automatic switch to stop, the tank overflows, right? Same with the body and food. You need a signal to tell you when you need to stop inserting fuel.

Leptin is also produced during sleep, and in combination with ghrelin, is a primary driver of metabolism. And if you're not getting enough sleep, you're not producing these hormones in the right amounts, so you lose the ability to properly regulate metabolism.

In the case of truckers, the shifts are irregular, and their schedules are compounded by time pressure. Thanks to these factors, truckers average only 4.78 hours of sleep per 24 hours. As a result, they're not producing the hormones to regulate metabolism properly. So the majority of drivers are not getting the signals that they need to eat. (The National Sleep Foundation recommends between 7 and 9 hours of sleep for the average adult, though about 43 percent of us get less than that on a regular basis.)

On the average, truckers eat only 2.6 times per day, often skipping entire meals, sometimes to the point that they're technically malnourished. But when they do eat, they often overeat. Why? Primarily as a function of hormones. They're not hungry because their ghrelin levels are low and they're not getting the signal that says *You're hungry and need to eat*. But they do eat, and they're not getting signaled that they need to stop, because their leptin levels are low. Because those hormones are produced in sleep and the truckers are sleep-deprived, their hormones are affected.

So sleep—not diet—is actually the root of the problem. Bottom line: you don't sleep properly, you're not going to regulate your food intake properly.

MY METABOLIC SLEEP ADVENTURE

When I first started tracking my sleep, I was getting around 6 hours and 15 minutes each night. My sleep scores—an index for the quality of sleep—were around 60 to 70 percent. The digital health technology told me exactly where I was on a scale from zero to optimal. It was then up to me to improve.

As I stated above, nearly half of us are chronically sleep deprived. But I don't want to be in this group, and I don't want to do *anything* in life at 60 to 70 percent of my potential. So then the question became, "If this is where I am, what do I have to do to get better?"

I read up on sleep hygiene and came up with ways to try to improve both the quality and quantity. This became clear first: I needed to "respect the sleep environment." This means different things for different people. For me, it meant reserving my bedroom for sleep. I didn't watch TV in there, didn't exercise in there. I wanted my mind and body to associate my bedroom with sleeping. *I'm here; now it's time to sleep.*

Next, I tried to block out all the light possible. I put up curtains and made sure that no lights—not even lights from the phone—were left on. As you know, I'm a huge advocate of technology—everywhere but the bedroom. I removed all electronic devices from my bedside. My alarm clock was battery powered.

Hard as it was, I even made sure to leave my cell phone far from the bed. Turns out, this is a big issue right now. (With no end in sight.) Researchers say that it's almost as though the smartphone is designed *ideally* to disrupt our sleep. Some of this is psychological. We all need to disengage when we sleep. But when your phone is within arm's reach as you sleep, you will still feel connected—to work, to your social life, to Facebook.

It's physiological, too, though. Melatonin is the hormone that promotes sleep; when you expose yourself to the light emitted by your smartphone, it inhibits melatonin.

Sleep is another example of your body being connected to your environment. The body picks up on signals from your surroundings. This isn't new. Before electricity, when the sun set and the temperatures cooled and atmospheric changes occurred at night, these all sent signals to our bodies to secrete serotonin and melatonin and signal that it was time to rest. Darkness was not conducive to human activity; it was conducive to sleeping!

If you want to get good at anything, what's the fastest and most effective way to achieve the goal? Do it consistently, build a routine. Same for sleeping. I realized that if I undertook the same routines and fell asleep at the same time every day, it would help. I power down my electronics about an hour before bedtime. I drink a small cup of chamomile tea. I read a book, but usually get through only a few pages before I am out.

Using a sleep tracker, I made sure to keep the same bedtime and then look at the data each week to let me know how I was doing. Same for waking up. If you rise at the same time, your body will crave the routine. So often we get up at the same time each day and soon discover our bodies don't even require the alarm clock.

Now, I sleep between 7.2 and 7.4 hours a night. My sleep onset latency is roughly 12 minutes—that is, I fall asleep and lose wakefulness 12 minutes after my head hits the bed. My sleep index is now more than 90 percent of optimal. Not perfect yet. But I'm still working on it.

BETTER METABOLISM THROUGH EXERCISE

If you exercise for sixty minutes at a moderate level, that long exertion over a long period has an effect on your serum ghrelin, triggering production of the hormone. This is why you feel famished after you, say, play a three-set tennis match or go for a long run. Studies will show, for example, that people who exercise for 50 minutes will burn an extra 200 to 300 calories, but they also eat an extra 200 to 300 calories.

On the other hand, when you exercise according to 4-Minute Fit, limiting yourself to no more than 15 minutes of working out, it's a short enough interval that it doesn't stimulate the production of ghrelin. You won't feel hungry. What's more, shorter, more intense workouts can affect your other hormones in ways that are going to make you sleep better. When you sleep better, you produce the correct levels of leptin and ghrelin, you regulate metabolism and hunger better, and then you eat better or more regularly, and that brings you back into harmony. It's a spiral of good effects.

To understand fully the benefits of vigorous activity, it is important to know this: there is a difference between weight-loss thinking and fat-loss thinking. Weight-loss thinking makes calorie-burning the goal.

Fat-loss thinking is all about hormones. Most people exercise because they believe that burning more calories is the way to lose weight. This is part of the "eat less, exercise more" approach.

But when we exercise more, the natural compensatory reaction of the body is to eat more, while also slowing the metabolic processes in other aspects of our daily lives, frustrating our weight-loss efforts. And when we exercise less, the body responds by suppressing appetite, which keeps our metabolism at a low level, further frustrating our weight-loss attempts. Again, this is due to the action of leptin and ghrelin. Leptin is produced in the fat cells: as soon as you start losing weight (fat), your falling leptin levels signal your body to start eating more and slow down your metabolic fat-burning, causing you to hold on to that fat.

Rising leptin levels do the opposite: they shut off hunger and stimulate metabolism. In normal-weight people, this works to maintain normal bodyweight—you gain a little fat, your leptin rises, signaling your body to stop eating so much.

However, in obese people, this mechanism often goes haywire. As we gain weight, our leptin levels increase. But if our metabolisms are already compromised—by a lack of sleep, by too many carbohydrates, by too much stress, or by unhealthy eating schedules—we continue to pack on pounds. When leptin levels are very high for long periods (which often coincides with obesity), leptin *resistance* sets in—the body no longer responds to the cue to stimulate metabolism. This means very high leptin levels can cause both increased hunger and slowed metabolism. This is the common perception of obese people—they just eat and eat and eat while their metabolism gets slower and slower.

Now, remember what we learned about mitochondria and the creation of ATP? When we use brief bouts of intense, muscle-producing exercise, we create a maximum demand for energy; the muscles are requiring so much energy that the mitochondria have to operate at full capacity. Meaning they have to use as much ATP as possible in as many cells as possible. The more muscles you use at maximum intensity, the greater the demand for ATP. And the body must create more and bigger mitochondria to answer that demand. Bam! You've just reset your metabolism.

> *Testimonial:* "YOU TELL ME IF IT WORKS"
>
> *One time I was standing in front of a mirror at a Petro truck stop in Nevada doing my exercises. To the side, to the side, kick your leg up. Just then another female trucker walked in, glared, walked out, and called the manager in to gripe. The manager came by but explained that I could use the mirror however I wanted. So the woman asks me, "What are you doing, anyway?"*
>
> *"My daily exercise," I said.*
>
> *"How's that work exactly?" she wondered, now getting curious.*
>
> *"I'm trying to stay healthy, doing the best I can, when I can," I said. "My heart rate will go up, and when I get back in the truck my metabolism will be a little higher."*
>
> *"Well, has it worked?" the woman asked.*
>
> *I told her I lost weight and cut down my medication for diabetes. I feel better and have more energy. I said, "Honey, you tell me if that sounds like it works." —Yvonne Johnson, nineteen-year-veteran truck driver*

THE METABOLISM "SPIKE"

I've talked a lot about the importance of "spiking" metabolism in the first few chapters. Now I've shown you how creating those metabolic spikes forces your body to create more and larger mitochondria, setting you up for a higher day-long metabolism and greater all-day calorie burn.

We track these metabolic spikes through a measurement called *metabolic equivalents*, or METs. One MET represents the amount of oxygen you consume and the number of calories you burn at rest. If you see, say, 7 METs on a treadmill, it represents your working 7 times as hard as you would be at rest, consuming 7 times as much oxygen, and burning 7 times as many calories as you would be at rest.

As a rule of thumb:

0 to 3 METs: light activity

3 to 6 METs: moderate activity

6 or more METs: vigorous activity

The people who don't exercise? Whose extent of bodily movement is easing in and out of a truck or getting in and out of their car at the office? They're only spiking their metabolism to just over 3 METs, maybe 4 if they're lucky and walk really fast.

So the people doing nothing, no exercise? Their METs are in sedentary position for the vast majority of the day, easily 23 hours, probably closer to 23:30. And it goes above the sedentary mark only when they walk, and even that yields only 3 or 4 METs, not even the middle of the moderate zone. This is a very slow, or low, metabolism. This will probably sound harsh, but they have the metabolism of a cow. Think about it: a cow or a slow-moving mammal that has a really low metabolism.

The people doing the four minutes of exercise? For those four minutes, their metabolism goes from 1 to a level in the 6+ range. That puts an incredible demand on their fat-burning system, sparking the need for more ATP. And, like many things in life, when you use it to its full potential, it adapts and grows and gets stronger—in this case, through the increase in mitochondria. So the person doing nothing isn't challenging his metabolism; the person doing four minutes of exercise is. If you're getting 6.3 METs one week, odds are good you'll work comparably hard and be at 6.4 METs the next week. Every week, you are improving your metabolism.

But just because you have more ATP, and a greater capacity to use it, you aren't necessarily going to produce more energy. You need to have enough of the proper fuel to produce that energy. And that's why the dietary component of this program—reducing carbs and boosting protein—is also essential.

THE METABOLIC CONSEQUENCE

At Prime, I studied how the lack of metabolic spikes affected drivers' body composition, looking at both male and female drivers, their ages, and their years of driving experience. The data shows that for men and women combined, the average BMI increases from 32.05 in the first sixty days of one's driving career and reaches a peak of 35.79 within three years. During this time, for men, their visceral fat rating— measure of the amount of fat surrounding the internal organs— increases from 14.7 in the first six months of driving to an average of 16.77 by the end of the third year. Consider: a visceral fat rating of 12 or less is considered normal and healthy.

For men, the older you are, the higher the average visceral fat rating, too. So if you start your driving career later in life, you are more likely to gain more abdominal fat in the first three years of driving. Male drivers between fifty-five and fifty-nine have the highest BMI of any age group (33.8), while female drivers between fifty-one and fifty-five have the highest BMI (35.93) for their gender's age group range. Visceral fat ratings for those groups are 17.95 and 11.38, respectively.

When you live a sedentary existence, as most of us are forced to do, just four minutes of vigorous activity a day can change your metabolic capacity. Without those four minutes, the consequences are inescapable.

THE PREMATURE DEATH EPIDEMIC

Statistics state that the average life-span of a long haul driver is just 61 to 64 years of age. What's happening to drivers?

Drivers BMI by Years of Service

Years of Service	# of Drivers	BMI
60 Days or Less	621	32.05
61 Days to 180 Days	812	32.02
181 Days to 1 Year	286	33.44
Over 1 Year to 3 Years	**304**	**35.79**
Over 3 Years to 5 Years	125	33.82
Over 5 Years	**171**	**35.10**

BMI by Age & by Gender

Male	# of Drivers	BMI
21 to 25	301	31.21
26 to 30	321	32.95
31 to 35	267	33.38
36 to 40	220	32.51
41 to 45	268	33.32
46 to 50	253	33.33
51 to 55	196	32.98
56 to 60	**141**	**33.85**
61 to 65	60	30.76
66 to 70	12	30.77
71 to 75	6	30.43
76 to 80	1	26.31

10 Stay Motivated for a Lifetime of Leanness

A goal without a plan is just a wish.

Entrepreneurs, champion athletes, and other successful people will usually agree that at some point they learned one critical lesson: the planning process is both the longest and the most important part of any project.

Ordinarily, people don't spend enough time planning. They may get a good—even a great—idea. They may catch a moment of excitement or motivation and then initiate some action. Then, after having taken a few steps but not the time to properly think it through, they get to a point where they don't know what the next step is. They might guess about the next step; they might be paralyzed by indecision. Instead of having figured out how it should go, they don't have the ability to stay on course because they don't know what or where the course is now.

If you plan out your next several weeks ahead of time, you'll avoid stepping into the same traps that undo so many people's best weight-loss intentions. This chapter will help you do that.

HOW TO "SEE" THE FUTURE

When I left Yale, I didn't have a plan. For me, that was a good thing. For the previous eleven years or so, I had been living according to a detailed plan—specifically, training to become a state swimming champion, getting a swim scholarship to college, becoming a collegiate champion, competing at the Olympic Trials, qualifying for the Olympic team.

Within that grand plan, there were plans. And plans within those plans. Until I left school, I never knew what it was like to wake up and *not* have a plan for the day ahead, not know what needed to be done and exactly how I was going to do it. There's a tremendous amount of value to living that way. It can virtually guarantee progress in the desired direction, and it leads to the consistent production of results.

This is great, so long as it allows room for other areas of life—rest and relaxation, fun and relationships. That has to be built into the plan, too. When a person starts to become obsessive to the point that negative or harmful effects can be observed, that's when the plan stops being healthy. That didn't happen in my case, at least not at first. But there were some observable negative effects, after I failed to qualify for the Olympic Trials in 1992. I was so goal oriented, so attached to a plan, that when I didn't achieve my goal—and questioned the plan I had been following so closely—it caused me to question a lot about how I was living my life. This led to one of the darkest periods I've ever experienced.

So when I left school with no plan, well, that was actually good for me, too. It provided some well-needed balance. When I failed to qualify for the 1992 Olympic Trials, I didn't want to swim anymore. My heart wasn't in it. And without swimming, without my identity as a great swimmer, I didn't feel too good about myself. And I didn't want to be around people. So I became withdrawn. I kept to myself. I didn't have much ambition or energy. I didn't care about graduating. Nothing seemed to make any sense. My attempted suicide was more a cry for attention and help than anything else.

I still managed to go to a few classes, and I was reading a book by the philosopher Søren Kierkegaard. He talked about making "a leap of faith." I realized that I was faced with a blank canvas for my life. I was free to choose the brush, the paint, the colors, and the brushstrokes to create a new vision, a new future for myself. So I was "lost" and didn't know what to do each morning when I woke up. So what? The question shifted from "What do I need to do today?" or "What's next on my schedule?" to "What do I want to do today?" More and more, the answer kept coming up, "I want to go surfing." It was time to make a leap of faith. So that's what I decided to do. It didn't matter that it was winter in New Haven, that I didn't have any money, that I didn't have a surfboard or know how to surf. What mattered was that *I decided*. Once I did that, it became simple. Where's the best place for me to go surfing right now? California, duh! How do I get there? Head west. Simple. I just started taking one step after another—get on a bus, go to the on ramp and stick my thumb out, ride in someone's car, repeat, until I reached Huntington Beach, got a surfboard, and started paddling out into the surf.

Likewise, it doesn't matter if you want to lose 80 pounds, you haven't exercised in ten years, and you haven't used your oven for the last three years. You just *decide* and then keep moving in the direction you want to go.

Interestingly, though, it wasn't long before I started working, serving in various causes and nonprofit organizations as a program developer, project planner, and grant writer. All my previous years of structuring plans, schedules, training programs, goals, implementation procedures, and so on helped develop a very valuable skill set that I began to realize lots of people didn't have.

The real value of a well-crafted plan is that once you embark on it, you can "see" what lies ahead. When challenges or opportunities come along, at least you have the plan as a source of orientation to determine what to do, if following some course of action is going to be of direct, of indirect, or of no benefit.

Here's an example. Before I enrolled in Prime's student driver program, I did my research and found out that, after all my truck expenses, I could reasonably expect to make an average of $900 per week. Then I calculated all my expenses and the cost of personal needs. Once I had my budget, I subtracted that from my weekly expected income and that's how much money I would have left over to put into savings. Then I calculated how much I could save each year. Optimistically, I calculated I could save $30,000 a year. So after a three-year lease, I could have $90,000 in the bank!

That became my goal. Each week, the first thing I did was to pay whatever bills and obligations I faced—food, my cell phone, truck note, et cetera. At the time, I was single. I would put $500 into savings. Whatever I had left over was considered "bonus" money that I could permit myself to use for anything I wanted. Having this plan firmly in place, I made sure that:

- ► my business (trucking) was functional

- ► my responsibilities were going to be met

- ► my goals were going to be met

At that point, there wasn't any doubt about succeeding—I *knew* I was going to succeed. All I had to do was execute the plan. Then, when someone asked me, "Hey, do you want to go here?" or "Do you want to buy this?" or "Do you want to invest in this?" I could say yes or no based on whatever leftover money I had. I never put the business, the responsibilities, or the goals in jeopardy of not being fulfilled. A solid, thought-out plan helps eliminate failure. Figuring out the details, the sequences, and the procedures can be as important as the execution.

I have taken what I've learned about the value of planning and incorporated it into 4-Minute Fit. It takes what would otherwise be a complicated plan and makes it simple. That plan then becomes simply to follow these seven strategies. Then each day it takes only a little bit of preparation to fulfill the seven strategies. I'm going to repeat them here, because as long as you keep them in mind, your path to success is clear:

The Seven Strategies

1. No matter what, get four minutes of exercise a day, and eventually increase that to fifteen minutes.

2. Each workout must include at least four minutes of vigorous activity.

3. Work multiple muscle groups at the same time.

4. Always eat after a workout.

5. Eat breakfast. Then eat something every three hours.

6. Keep healthy snacks within reach.

7. Log your nutrition and fitness.

But I encourage you to develop your own plan within my plan. For a short-term plan, ask yourself each day:

- What do I anticipate eating today?

- When do I anticipate eating my meals?

- What will I do to try to meet my nutritional goals?

- When do I anticipate doing my workout?

- When I do my workout, where will I be and how will that influence the exercises I choose?

- If something comes up, what is my backup plan?

Plans are subject to change. Plans are designed to be flexible. But between my plan and your plan, we should have a road map for where we're going. As you create your plan for success, keep in mind a line often attributed to Ben Franklin: "By failing to prepare, you are preparing to fail."

UNDERSTAND YOUR PHYSICAL AND MENTAL CYCLES

Everything in nature exists as part of a cycle. Our solar system is based on a 24,000-year cycle. We have lunar cycles. We have the cycle of four seasons; a cycle of twelve months; a weekly seven-day cycle. We have our circadian rhythms, which comprise our daily cycle, connecting our physiology to the environment.

Similar to our circadian rhythms, we have a cycle that I identify as biorhythms. Consider a wave: there is a point where we reach a peak, then we come back to normal, then we reach a valley. So much in our lives resembles this.

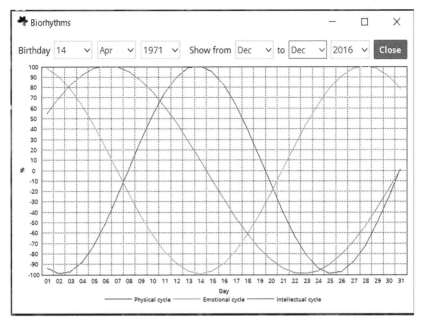

Siphiwe's Bio Well biorhythm chart for December 2016

That's why, on some days, your workout seems easy; on others, it's a slog to get through. On some days, you're a little tired and unfocused no matter how much sleep you got the night before; on others, you burn through the day with startling efficiency.

How do we learn about our rhythms? Simple answer: the *digital health devices* that I keep harping on. (Forgive me. But, really, they work wonders.) Ours is the first generation in which the average person has the capacity and ability to monitor and measure these cycles. This really gives us a measure of true power and control over our health.

As I write this, I am using a device called Bio-Well. It's a combination of Western technology and Eastern traditional medicine. It works on the theory that every part of the body is connected to every other part of the body and measures the electron emissions coming off your fingertip. Taking snapshots of the energy off your fingertips, it diagnoses the energy systems in your body and then, using sophisticated algorithms, figures out your biorhythm cycle. You then take that information and plan your day (or week or month or even year) accordingly.

I learned about these cycles the hard way. In 2015, I visited with my swim coach, Gary Hall Sr. He provided me with a series of workouts and said, "Look, Siphiwe, if you want to win the Masters Swimming World Championships in 2017, you have to increase your training volume." I had been training three times per week for one hour; he said I had to increase that to six practices a week. When a three-time Olympic medalist and former world record holder in five events gives you a plan, you take it seriously. I went from three practices a week to five and then to six. I also added strength training.

One problem: I upgraded this training the very week that my biorhythms said I was in a physical low. I lost my voice—which didn't help my speaking engagement I had that week—and became sick. Looking back, I had increased my training at a physical valley, precisely the wrong time. And I paid the price, coming down with a respiratory infection, which caused me to miss five days of practice.

Had I been paying attention, I could have said: "Hmm, my coach said that I need to increase my training from three days to six days. But I'm going to wait two weeks to do it when I'm physically at my best and better able to handle the load. Plus, I have this speaking engagement coming up, and that usually takes a lot out of me, so because I'm in a low cycle, now is not the time to do that."

Now? I take readings every morning. It takes me about five minutes to perform a scan. I can look at the data and within two minutes I can see what my biorhythms are. I've learned that the physical cycle has its own frequency; so do the intellectual cycle and the emotional cycle. Some days they will be in sync with each other. Those are special days.

You think back in history and wonder what role these cycles

played. When Michael Phelps or Usain Bolt wins a gold medal, were their physical, intellectual, and emotional peaks in harmony? I assume so. (If you're competing in the Olympics, you're definitely hoping for this.) Same for scientists when they made groundbreaking discoveries. What about actors who nail their auditions for big roles?

On the days when you don't have this synchronicity? Well, it's good to be prepared that it could be a "valley day" and not a "peak day." It doesn't mean those will be bad days; just that they might be suboptimal. And you can prepare: if you know your emotional cycle is at a low, that's probably not the day you want to call somebody to deal with a controversial subject or a delicate topic in your romantic relationship.

This technology is incredible—and it's only going to become more targeted and accurate. Imagine you're a CEO with a busy schedule. You're trying to manage all your appointments and obligations and travel with fitness and balanced nutrition and speaking engagements. Wouldn't you want to use a device that tells you about the optimal and suboptimal times of the day? That knows some of the triggers that can make you sick? That makes you more efficient while mitigating the risk of your coming down with an illness because of exhaustion?

One warning: it's easy to become fanatical about the cycles. There's a science that combines qigong (basically a Chinese holistic system) with these biorhythms that supposedly enables you to know every cycle for every hour of the day. Some people get to the point where they can't do anything until there's perfect alignment. That is going too far with it. At some point trying the "game the system" becomes counterproductive.

On the other hand, consider this. All business, and particularly business *owners*, are concerned with productivity and *maximizing* productivity. I have a device called the Readiband (by Fatigue Science) that tracks my sleep and circadian cycles and calculates my mental effectiveness score. "Peak" mental effectiveness is a score over 90. Now, as an employer, do I want employees at work with mental effectiveness scores in the 60s or 70s, or do I want my employees in the 90s? What if each year my evaluation included how much time I spent at work in the peak zone and what my average mental effectiveness score was for the year? What if I were incentivized based on improving my peak mental effectiveness at work, which would mean getting better sleep and nutrition? What if I could prove to my boss that I could be more productive with a shorter workday allowing me better sleep and higher mental effectiveness?

Bottom line: If you invest in the technology that helps you to monitor your cycles, you'll know a lot more about what your body and mind are up to. If getting the most out of both is important to you, this is one way to reach that goal. But also tap into your body and be wise about when you push yourself.

DO IT FOR THE MONEY

Most of us are motivated by money. It impacts our decision-making in all sorts of ways. When we talk about making "rational" choices, it usually means making choices that are in our economic or financial best interests. And for most of us, the pain of losing a dollar is more powerful—and more of a motivation—than the pleasure we get from winning a dollar.

This concept is known as *loss aversion*. In a famous psychology experiment, subjects are given two gambles with identical payoffs and odds, but they are framed differently. In the first gamble, they're told that there will be a coin flip. "If it lands on heads, you get one hundred dollars. If it's tails, you get nothing."

In the second gamble, they are first given a hundred-dollar bill to hold. Then they are told, "We're going to flip a coin. If it lands on heads, you can keep the money. It's yours. But if it lands on tails you have to pay back the hundred dollars. Hand it over."

It's the same proposition in both scenarios, right? A 50-50 chance for the person to make one hundred dollars.

But subjects dislike the second experiment much more than the first—even though the actual gains and losses are identical. Why is this? Because in the second experiment, there is a perceived loss. They have that hundred-dollar bill in their hands and 50 percent of the time (that is, when the coin flip is heads) they experience the sting of loss, the pain of having to give up something. This is loss aversion.

We see it in all sorts of ways. Marketing and advertising execs cater to this bias. They know that telling customers they'll avoid a surcharge is more effective than advertising a rebate. Would you rather get a five-dollar discount or avoid a five-dollar surcharge? A study of insurance policies, for instance, found that price increases had twice the effect on customer switching, compared to price decreases. Again, we like gains. But not as much as we hate loss.

A pair of Yale psychologists used this concept with dieting. Both wanting to lose weight, they saw shows like *The Biggest Loser* and watched people get rewarded for losing weight. They wondered: *What if, instead of motivating ourselves with rewards, we tried to motivate with fear of loss?* They made a bet with each other that didn't involve reward but punishment: If they didn't lose weight, they would have to pay the other $1,000.

Within two years, the professors didn't see a dime of the other's money—and they had lost eighty pounds between them. They even started a company based on the principle to help people lose weight and achieve other personal goals. If you don't live up to your end of the contract, they give your money to charity or a designated beneficiary. (Another more severe variation: the losers have to donate the money to a cause that runs counter to their political sensibilities; gun haters contributing to the NRA, pro-lifers contributing to Planned Parenthood.)

Another concept from psychology is called *effort justification*. It basically says that when we make sacrifices to pursue a goal, we elevate the attractiveness of that goal. In other words, the more we struggle and suffer to achieve something, the more value we put on it. The more brutal the fraternity and sorority hazing, the more loyalty its members are likely to show. The more we work and sweat to build something—say, a piece of Ikea furniture—the more we value that item. When we pay for access to a gym, we are more likely to use it than when we are given access to the same gym for free. Which is to say that we are struggling (by paying our hard-earned money), and as a result we value the opportunity more.

In my program, I use both principles—loss aversion and effort justification—to try to get people to change their behavior. Here's how Prime does it. We charge a fee of $400 for entry, but we dangle this carrot: if you complete the program, you get your $400 back. The looming specter of loss, of losing that four hundred bucks, will hopefully be another motivation not to quit. The way I look at it: those unwilling to put "skin in the game" are showing that they are not ready for behavior change.

I also don't avoid the reality that improving your health and lifestyle can be a struggle. It's hard work. It really is. But by stressing this, by making people feel like they are really exerting themselves to achieve their goals, I'm hopeful they'll value the experience and be less likely to put the weight back on or slip back into unhealthy habits.

DO IT FOR YOUR INNER CHILD

Early on, there was a driver we'll call John who enrolled in my program and was doing great at the start. After four weeks of a thirteen-week program, John was losing weight, getting in shape, changing his metabolism. He was nearly one-third of the way through, and I was confident that he was not only going to finish the program but be a top performer.

All of a sudden, I noticed that John had stopped exercising and logging his food altogether. *What?* My radar went off, and I called him. "John, I'm noticing that you're not putting in the work this week. What's going on, friend?"

"Well," he said, "I was in South Dakota, it was ten degrees out, and I was worried that if I worked out outdoors, I'd get sick."

I thought about it for a second. "That sounds reasonable," I said. "But when you realized that it wasn't healthy to work out outside, why didn't you go with the next best alternative? Why did you let the weather stop you? Go inside. Or work out inside of your truck. Or wait till you reach the next truck stop. You had all sorts of possibilities!"

I tried to impress upon him that if you're really committed to a goal, you work not to let challenges become roadblocks. There's a saying I'm quite fond of: "When faced with a challenge, the committed heart seeks a solution. The uncommitted heart seeks an escape." We talked a bit more. And finally the real reason came out: John confessed that he didn't want anyone looking at him.

Aha, now we're getting somewhere. I said: "So it wasn't really about the weather. It was about your being embarrassed or feeling shame."

"That's right. I know myself, and if someone said something negative or mocking to me, it would have really upset me."

It was clear that this was lodged in his subconscious, like so many of our thoughts are. And it wasn't until we talked about it that he was *consciously* linking his painful childhood experiences to his decision to quit exercising. But now that the issue was out there in the open, I kept pressing.

"But why would you let someone else prevent you from achieving your goals? Who is this person who's so important to you—whose name you don't know; who you might not ever see again—to whom you're giving so much power? I bet that something happened to you in childhood that you're still dealing with. And it's not just stopping you from losing weight, but it's stopping you from doing a lot of other things."

"That's right," he said. "In second grade, I was a chubby kid. Whenever I had to do things in front of the class, other kids laughed at me or made fun of me."

I wouldn't have known it just from looking at the data and the logs. But having a discussion with John made it clear why he had suddenly stopped the program. And, having discussed it, he promised to address it, which he did.

What I also didn't know at the time: John's situation would come up frequently in my face-to-face consultations with drivers. There is often a negative event from childhood that has carried over to adulthood and plays a huge role in lowering self-esteem. And as a result, drivers have built up and reinforced this behavior mechanism that makes them avoid being seen and fearful of what other people might think of them.

The problems, of course, perpetuate themselves. You don't want to do activities outside or in front of other people and guess what? You become less active. You then become bigger and less healthy and feel worse about yourself and guess what? You're only going to be less likely to undertake activities in front of others or risk any kind of mockery. It's a cascading, vicious cycle.

I'm not a psychologist or a counselor, but I have an antidote for this. My standard approach: I simply ask folks, "Do you want to let that experience from second grade continue to diminish or even destroy your life, or not? You have a choice. You can focus and speculate on the negative, this person—real or imagined—who might mock you. You can choose to invest negative energy on this possibility. Or you can choose to say, 'For every person who's doing that, there's also the person I am *inspiring*. When they see me going out there, at three hundred fifty pounds and doing my jumping jacks, doing the best I can at genuinely trying to better myself, they are going to be motivated."

You're out there exercising, maybe looking a little goofy. But I guarantee this: Someone will see the choice you've made. And then will say to himself, *If that person can do it, why can't I?* When you're wrestling with yourself—to work out or not to work out?—think about this person, not the person who might be mocking you. Get into the subconscious and reengineer it to get the behavior you want.

Obviously, there's a lot of complexity here. People spend years in counseling before they can access the subconscious. I don't mean for this chapter to minimize the effects of bullying, traumatic childhood experiences, or learned childhood behavior that stifles development. I don't overlook the courage it can take to step out of your comfort zone, to leave yourself vulnerable, to risk rekindling painful memories.

But much of what I do is not about the science of weight loss, but about the science of behavior change—and perhaps that is another book. And I have seen that once we address the subconscious, we have so much power in our choices. In this case, you either can take care of your own health, fitness, and, ultimately, happiness. Or you can give in to the haters and the mockers. The choice is yours.

DO IT FOR AMERICA

Again, let's be clear: We are a nation at war against an enemy that's infiltrating us from the inside. It's attacking our personal financial well-being and destroying our health, but it's doing the same to our country. It's time for us all to realize that we owe it to ourselves, to our families, and to America to take a stand and fight back. Here's a new way to look at the obesity crisis: in addition to improving your health and fitness for your own purposes, you're also doing it for your country.

It might sound crazy at first. And I'm not saying that the 150 million-plus Americans who are overweight are also unpatriotic. But think about it: our obesity epidemic comes at a huge cost to the United States health-care system. According to the Centers for Disease Control, we spend $150 billion every year to treat obesity-related illness. (And that's a 2014 figure; the number is supposed to double by the end of the decade.) That comes at a huge expense to the nation. We're talking about a preventable condition that is soaking the United States for almost $500 million a day!

What's more, according to Columbia University's School of Public Health, workplace absenteeism in the United States linked to obesity-related diseases—diabetes and heart disease, among others—costs $8.65 billion a year, almost $1 billion in California alone. Again, huge numbers and a huge blow for the American economy.

When I work with a truck driver whom I know will respond to this patriotic tack, my speech goes something like this:

"You love America, right? It's the best country on earth, right? Well, then, shouldn't you be willing and able to make a small sacrifice? In the past, when America has been at war or in a crisis, the citizens have been asked to make sacrifices. Sometimes it was rationing food items. Sometimes it was sending care packages to soldiers overseas. Other times, it was your patriotic duty to buy war bonds.

"It may not be conventional combat, but we're in a war against obesity. Without question, it's a national crisis. That is one rare issue that political leaders agree on, regardless of party. We can barely staff an army and a national reserve because of this problem. The US Department of Defense must recruit nearly 190,000 new military personnel every year to replace those retiring or leaving military service for other reasons. Nearly one-quarter of all new applicants to the military are medically disqualified because of excessive weight and body fat. (Disqualification due to obesity ranks far higher than the second-top reason: smoking marijuana.)

"The military also estimates that more than two-thirds of America's youth would fail to qualify for military service because of physical, behavioral, or educational shortcomings. The biggest issue? Obesity. Think about it: the strength of the nation's future military—the greatest in the world—is being imperiled because of obesity.

"What's being asked of you? Not much. *Just four minutes of vigorous exercise each day.* It doesn't matter when. Devote that time after you brush your teeth and before your morning shower. Knock out those four minutes on a lunch break or before dinner.

"But if everyone who was obese could make that small sacrifice, it would mark a huge turning point in this national crisis. Think about how much more efficient and productive American industry would be. Think about how much stronger the health-care system could be. Think about all the better ways in which that $150 billion in US health-care costs could be used. Again, do it for yourself. But do it for your country, too."

DO IT FOR THE REST OF US

As hard as it is to build consensus among politicians, as deeply divided as this country can be on social issues, here's a rare point of commonality: obesity is serious business. It affects everything from the economy to health-care costs to the military. Sociologists talk about the cost it has on corporate culture and productivity. Teachers talk about the negative impact it has on education. Economists talk about how it strains our economy through health-care costs and takes a toll on national spending. We talk about obesity as a national crisis. We talk about this "war on obesity." Well, if it's that big an epidemic—and if it's not only a war, but a winnable war—why are we not doing more?

Here's a thought exercise: what is to stop us from starting a national movement devoted to health and fitness?

- ▶ In schools all over the country, classes say the Pledge of Allegiance each morning. That's great. But what if, after the pledge, teachers said, "We're now going to continue our patriotic duty and take four minutes to be active"?

- ▶ What if every company said, "It can be before your shift or after your shift, but every employee has to devote four minutes a day to exercise to turn up your metabolism so we're burning fat while at our desks"?

- We have all sorts of requirements before students graduate from high school or college. *You have to have proficiency in a foreign language. You have to have a certain skill level in math or science.* Why not add that you have to have a certain fitness level, or you have to have a BMI under 30?

- What if there were some sort of bipartisan commission made up of all kinds of doctors, physiologists, physical trainers, psychologists, and workplace experts tasked with coming up with a national exercise plan that everyone can do, at any point in the day, that requires no equipment and can be achieved in a few minutes? Then everything from public service commercials to free tracking apps could be used to encourage Americans to adopt this plan.

- We have public service ads (PSAs) for everything from anti-smoking to anti-gambling. Where are the PSAs telling us not to drink so much soda or why it's important to read nutritional labels or that four minutes of vigorous exercise has this host of benefits? If we're dealing with an epidemic, wouldn't we want to do a better job using mass communications to publicize solutions?

Again, this is a preventable problem, a reversible crisis, a winnable war. We should be asking ourselves why aren't we, as a country, doing more?

But then again, we are doing more. We spend more on nutrition supplements, gym memberships, fitness gadgets and gizmos, etc. Yet the obesity epidemic gets worse. What we haven't done is come up with a single national movement that crystallizes, concentrates, and galvanizes the public in a simple, observable *course of action*. This course of action, I propose: the 4-Minute Movement. And of all the possible courses of actions to rally around, why this one? Because I have shown that it is the most effective, least time-consuming way to lose weight, one that has actually worked for the unhealthiest occupation in America.

Afterword

When I started my Fitness Trucking program, my goals were humble: I wanted to help myself, and I wanted to help the men and women I worked with every day—people who were sick, struggling, ashamed, in danger, and desperate.

What I believe I've created, however, is the beginning of a movement.

More and more of us have begun to realize that short, intense workouts—workouts you can fit into any schedule and work around any constraints—can and will change your life. In spring of 2016, the *Wall Street Journal* reported that there were more than 700 health and fitness apps in the Apple store, double the amount from 2014. And a study in the journal *PLOS ONE* found that doing just three workouts a week of ten minutes each—with only one minute of high-intensity exercise per workout—was enough to stimulate "physiological changes linked to improved health in overweight adults."

But exercise is, at best, perhaps 20 percent of the equation. The real benefits of brief, intense workouts come from the growth of mitochondria, and that growth can't happen unless you're properly fueling your body all day long. 4-Minute Fit isn't just about four minutes of exercise; it's about taking four minutes every three hours to ensure your body's metabolism is getting the fuel it needs.

You have the power and the tools now to go from "I should" to "I did."

All you need is four minutes a day.

Index

accidents: of truck drivers, 111, 112
action plan: for fitness, 26–29
adipokines, 36, 38, 112
adiponectin, 13
adrenal glands, 60–61
Aerobics and Fitness Association of
America (AFAA), 18
Africa: Baleka's visit to, 6
Age and Ageing journal, 40
Agriculture Department, U.S. (USDA),
104
Alzheimer's, 40
American Heart Association, 37, 106
American Journal of Clinical Nutrition,
126, 171
analgesics, 68
angiotensinogen, 38
appetite
and junk food cycle, 110
See also hunger
Appetite magazine, 126
apps, 207. *See also* technology; *specific
app*
arthritis, 39
ATP (adenosine triphosphate), 70, 110,
176, 181–82, 184

Bacon, Travis (testimonial), 24
Bacteroidetes bacteria, 114
Baleka, Siphiwe
aha moment for, 9–10
awards and honors for, 2, 4, 15
"bonking" of, 154
childhood and youth of, 2–3
financial affairs of, 5–6, 10–11
motivation of, 188–92, 194
and Olympics, 2, 3, 4, 15, 188,
194–95
planning by, 188–92
as Prime in-house fitness coach,
31–32
renaming of, 6
self-image of, 7–8, 188–89
as single parent, 169
sinus problems of, 150–51
sleep adventure of, 178–80
and swimming, 2, 3–4, 5, 7, 11, 15,
188–89, 194
travels of, 5, 6, 150
as truck driver, 1, 6–9, 13–16,
151
See also specific topic
bananas, 124, 128, 160

belly fat
    and brain, 39–40
    cycle of, 112–13
    and gender, 184–85
    and GI tract, 113–14
    and metabolism, 35, 36, 112, 113,
        184–85
    and protein, 37, 40, 113–14, 126
    and quality of life, 40–41
    and stress, 142
    and tracking and mastering
        nutrition, 126
    See also specific topic
Bench Jumps (exercise), 93
Berardi, John, 158
Bicycle Crunches (exercise), 95–96
The Biggest Loser (TV show), 197
Bio-Well device, 193–94
biorhythms, 192–96
Bird Dogs (exercise), 91
blood pressure, 13, 38, 45, 69, 111
blood sugar, 37, 38, 45, 118, 154, 164
BMI (body mass index), 41, 41*n*, 111,
    184–85, 205
body fat
    and benefits of HIIT, 69, 70
    distribution of, 35–36
    and junk food cycle, 110
    late-night eating and, 133
    stress and, 142
    See also belly fat; fat burning; fat
        storage; *specific topic*
Bolt, Usain, 195
bones, 39
brain
    and belly fat, 39–40
    and distracted eating, 172
    junk food cycle and, 110
    and managing hunger, 163, 164,
        165
    stress and, 143
    and using food to spike
        metabolism, 158
bread: and good and bad food, 155

breakfast, 106, 128, 129, 132, 153,
    157–60, 191
breathing, hard, 21
brushing teeth
    as alternative to smoking, 147
    and stress analogy, 145
Burpees (exercise), 87–88

calcium, 108
calories
    and belly fat, 37
    burning of, 175–76
    counting, 127–28, 156
    daily consumption of, 127–29
    and exercise, 50, 176, 180–81
    and food log, 121
    and 4-Minute Fit, 48, 49, 127–28
    and good and bad food, 155
    importance of, 159
    late-night eating and, 133
    liquid, 104, 154–55
    and metabolism, 157, 158, 176,
        180–81, 183
    and muscles, 59
    obesity and, 107
    and protein, 126–27
    sex and, 168
    and smoking, 146
    in soda, 104
    and tracking and mastering
        nutrition, 126–28
    and weight gain, 103, 153
    and weight-loss/fat-loss thinking,
        180–81
Campanis, Al, 3
carbohydrates
    and belly fat, 38, 112, 113–14
    cardio training and, 59
    and cheating, 128–29
    cutting, 123–25, 129–30, 133
    daily consumption of, 123, 129–30,
        131
    and distracted eating, 172
    and eating after workouts, 160–61

exercise and, 21–22, 181
and food/nutrition log, 121, 129–30, 131
and good and bad food, 154–55
and junk food cycle, 109
late-night eating and, 133
and managing hunger, 164, 165, 167
metabolism and, 158, 159, 160–61, 181, 184
and oatmeal, 106
obesity and, 107
prevalence of, 104–5
as reason for weight gain, 14, 104–5
sources of, 104, 113, 124
and tracking and mastering nutrition, 118, 123–25, 127–28
cardio training, 59–61, 70
Cell journal, 50
Cell Metabolism journal, 37
Centers for Disease Control and Prevention (CDC), 9, 202
cheating, 128–29
childhood experiences: and motivation, 199–202
China: national fitness movement in, 28–29
cholesterol, 37–38, 45, 69, 106, 111, 118, 142
circadian rhythms, 160, 175–76, 196
City University of New York (CUNY), 49–50
cognitive restructuring, 18, 19, 117–18
cold baths, 68
colleagues: partnering with, 172
Columbia University, 39, 202
competition: and workouts, 61–63
consequences
and Goals Consequence Worksheet, 140, 141
and good and bad food, 156
and lack of metabolic spikes, 184–85

and motivation, 139–40
of stress, 144
consistency, 58, 132
See also routine
convenience, 17–18, 118
corporate wellness programs, 31–32
cortisol, 13, 61, 108, 109, 110, 142, 143
costs. *See* money; *specific cost*
cravings, food, 108, 112, 128, 143, 165–66, 167, 177
creating a metabolism-spiking 15-minute workout, 50–51
Cronometer, 119
Crunches (exercise), 90
CT (computed tomography) scans study, 39–40
cycle
belly fat, 112–13
of junk food, 108–11
understanding physical and mental, 192–96
of weight loss, 108–12

death, premature, 185
decision making
and motivation, 189, 196
and stress, 143
Defense Department, U.S. (DOD), 203
Devor, Steven T., 69
diabetes
and belly fat, 36–37, 38, 39, 40, 114
and DKA, 27
and good and bad food, 154
junk food cycle and, 108
as obesity-related disease, 13, 202
soda and, 115
and testimonial about 4-Minute Fit, 27
and understanding metabolism, 182
Diabetes Care, 115

About the Authors

Siphiwe Baleka is the founder of Fitness Trucking, LLC and serves as the driver health and fitness coach at Prime Inc., a commercial trucking company based in Springfield, Missouri. His innovative, on-the-go wellness program has helped thousands of truck drivers lose weight and reclaim their health. Formerly, Baleka served as the driver health editor for both *RoadKing* and *The Trucking Network* magazines. He graduated from Yale University and is the first African American named to the All-Ivy League swim team.

L. Jon Wertheim is the executive editor of *Sports Illustrated*, a sports television commentator for various networks, and author or coauthor of ten previous books, including *New York Times* bestsellers *Scorecasting* and *You Can't Make This Up*. He lives in New York City.